1 MONTH OF
FREE
READING

at

www.ForgottenBooks.com

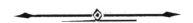

By purchasing this book you are eligible for one month membership to ForgottenBooks.com, giving you unlimited access to our entire collection of over 1,000,000 titles via our web site and mobile apps.

To claim your free month visit:

www.forgottenbooks.com/free838739

ISBN 978-0-483-49636-1
PIBN 10838739

THE KANSAS CITY

MEDICAL JOURNAL.

FEBRUARY, 1873.

Lecture on the Clinical Examination of Children.

By D. N. KINSMAN, A. M., M. D., Professor of Diseases of Women and Children, Starling Medical College, Columbus, Ohio.

Patience and care are required in the clinical examination of sick children. They cannot talk in most instances, and you must learn to read the *sign language* of disease.

This language is at once clear and explicit, as well as truthful, a statement which we cannot make, without very decided modifications, concerning the oral description of symptoms by adults.

When once you have learned to appreciate the objective signs or symptoms of disease, among children, you will delight more in the investigation of their diseases than those of adults. They are easily frightened, and this disorders circulation and respiration, hence you cannot commence the examination of a sick child abruptly upon your entrance into its room. There are, however, many things which you can study without contact with the child while it is becoming accustomed to your presence. You can observe the color of the skin. This is waxy in atrophy, tuberculosis and wasting diseases; yellow in icterus and post-natal discoloration. There are irregular patches of purplish hue in meningitis, dependent upon diminished power of the vaso-motor nerves; these are produced on the cheek, forehead and neck by pressure of the pillow or the nurse's arm. There is a general congestion of the face in some cases of typhoid fever in its early stages. A circumscribed patch is seen on the cheek in pneumonia and in hectic fever dependent upon tuberculosis or collections of pus. In pneumonia the patch is livid, in hectic, pink. The skin is leaden in color or blue in chills, livid in croup, capillary bronchitis, œdema of the lungs, and all diseases of imperfect aeration of the blood. A similar color is seen in cyanosis from whatever cause. There is paleness in nausea and shock. The "tache cérébrale," which is deemed pathognomonic of meningitis by Trousseau, may be brought out by a simple scratching of the skin, by the finger nail or a pencil. This is dependent upon the same cause as the irregular mottling of the cheek above described. Vogel attaches no value whatever to this sign, but I have seen it brought out in all its characteristics on numerous patients. The redness to which this name is applied persists for a considerable time after the application of the irritation, and I have never been able to produce it except in meningeal inflammation. There is also the white stripe, which may be produced upon the skin by similar means in scarlatina. There are also peculiar eruptions, which you will learn to recognize, in scarlatina, measles, erysipelas and variola.

The rose-colored spots of typhoid fever, the petechiæ of typhus, scorbutus, and epidemic cerebro-spinal meningitis, are often of great value in directing to a correct diagnosis.

In chronic diarrhœa the skin becomes of an earthy hue.

In cases of sudden fever from various causes the skin in children, after the lapse of hours, becomes covered with sudamina. These are caused by a restoration of cutaneous exhalation; the fluid cannot escape through the scarf skin and it accumulates beneath, raising it in the form of minute vesicles. This symptom is of no importance, except that it shows a relaxation of the skin, and an attempt on the part of nature to resume a normal function, which has for a time been arrested.

The eyes of a child when asleep, in health, are directed upward beneath the upper lid, and the pupils are evenly contracted. The pupils may be dilated, irregular or sluggish in their action from cerebral disease, or from disease located in the structure of the eye itself. They are often dilated to a great extent in the early stage of typhoid fever, and when this occurs it shows that the nervous system is profoundly implicated. Dilation occurs also in the later stages of diarrhœas, when there is great exhaustion. The eyelids are also partially open during sleep, in the later stages of exhausting diseases, as the result of loss of muscular tonicity in the orbicularis muscles. In the same cases there is an accumulation of sebaceous matter over the cornea, and a great loss of sensibility, for flies may crawl over the eye without any apparent inconvenience. These symptoms are indicative of great danger.

There is photophobia in meningeal or cerebral disease, also in phlyctenular conjunctivitis. Tears make their appearance about the fourth month, they disappear during severe disease, and their reappearance is an indication of improvement.

Respiration in diseases of the lungs becomes more frequent. The normal rate of respiration in children, when asleep and at rest, is about thirty per minute; when awake it sometimes rises as high as eighty per minute. The mere rate of respiration, since it is subject to so great variation, is not of any special symptomatic value. Respiration, however, is interrupted in cerebral disease and is a symptom of great value. In croup inspiration is noisy, in asthma and emphysema expiration is noisy. Respiration is sighing and slow in nausea.

Cough is another symptom to be referred to the respiratory organs. It is hoarse and ringing in the commencement of croup, becoming extinguished as the disease advances; spasmodic and subintrant in pertussis; constant and synchronous with each expiration in some cases of irritation of the laryngeal nerves.

Cough sometimes exists as a symptom of worms in the intestines, and of jaundice; in these cases it is of reflex origin.

The cry of children has been minutely studied by Billard, and, while I cannot subscribe to all he has written upon the subject, there are two cases in which the cry has diagnostic value. Skoda, I think, first clearly pointed out the difference of the cries in the delirium of typhoid fever and cerebro-spinal meningitis. In typhoid fever the cries are those of constantly changing fancies, and may be changed by external impressions, while in meningitis the cry is a constant repetition of the same word, at intervals more or less regular, with an unvarying cadence.

There are also a class of symptoms belonging to the motor system. The movements of the hand to the head, the ear, the mouth, the throat, are indications of disturbance in the several localities mentioned.

In some cases of cerebral irritation and typhoid fever I have observed that the hands are kept constantly in contact with the genitals, and I have learned to regard it as a grave symptom, and that to a great extent it is involuntary.

Jactitation occurs sometimes towards the close of exhausting diseases.

The persistent flexion of one extremity points to lesion in the brain. Flexion of the thumbs or toes, contractions of the eye-brows, grinding of the teeth and startings are often the prodromes of general convulsion. Contraction of the lower extremities, with crying, writhing and twisting of the body are symptoms of the colic, vesical irritation, rectal tenesmus, pricking of pins, etc., and a constant pulling at the penis in young boys, some-times is seen in calculous disorders, and in congenital phymosis.

There is retraction of the head in meningeal disease, irregu-lar muscular contraction without loss of consciousness in cho-rea, boring of the head into the pillow in cerebral irritation and rachitis.

Apathy and quietude in a child are suggestive of rachitis when there are no other indications of disease, and when this is joined to sweating about the head and general soreness, the diagnosis is positive.

Nearly all the above symptoms may be made out without touching the child, and many of them can be ascertained with-out waking it, if it is asleep, and you should never wake a child till you have noted the pulse, respiration and temperature, if you find it asleep.

The frequency and force of the pulse in young children has not the value for us that it has in the case of adults. It is very difficult for us to ascertain the average. An intermittent pulse points with great certainty to disease of the brain, and an ex-tremely frequent and feeble pulse is the forerunner of dissolu-tion.

With the digestive organs many symptoms of value are con-nected. Vomiting may be incidental to the conformation of the stomach, or a symptom of disease. It is one of the first symp-toms of scarlatina, variola or intussusception; it accompanies abdominal inflammations, whooping cough, and sometimes pneumonia. It is one of the most rebellious symptoms of meningeal inflammation; in this disease it is forcible, and has been compared to the action of a force pump. The abdomen is tumid and distended in diarrhœa, but retracted and boat-shaped in meningitis. It fluctuates in dropsy and purulent collections in the peritoneal cavity, is nodular from enlargement of mesenteric glands. In cases of intussusception the coils of the intestines roll beneath the surface like a mass of writhing snakes.

The stools should be carefully examined, for from them you can often derive indications for treatment.

The presence of undigested masses of casein or other albuminous matter tells you the disorder is in the stomach digestion. Excessive watery discharges in summer point to sympathetic paralysis. Worms and their ova will also indicate to you the necessity for their expulsion.

Examine the mouth and fauces, for evidence of disease, for it is in this locality where we commonly first recognize the presence of pseudo-membranous and diphtheritic deposits. The urine should be examined for sugar, albumen and urinary deposits; also for casts of tubes and renal and vesical epithelium.

There are many things to be learned by inspection, and in obscure troubles it should never be neglected. Needles have been found driven into the brain through the fontanelles, perforating the chest and the abdomen, and plunged into the liver.

One of the earliest evidences of diseased action is found in variations of temperature. The mean temperature of newly born children is a little less, say one-half a degree, than in adults. In scleremia there is a reduced temperature from the beginning.

The production of heat in excess of the natural standard is the result of several factors. There may be increased metamorphosis of tissues; impressions upon the vaso-motor nerves, and the action of poisons upon the blood, as in zymotic diseases, where we infer an action similar to a ferment—all these may be capable of modifying the heat-producing processes; but the subject as yet is to be more fully investigated before we can be fully enlightened. This much we know, there seems to be a fully established law that according to the height of the temperature above 98.40 (Fah.), the gravity of the case and its danger is increased. Adults may have a range of twelve degrees. In children, Roger has recorded oscillations amounting to over eighteen degrees. In intermittent fever there is a great rise of temperature during the febrile paroxysm, often to 104° or 106°, but it speedily begins to decline. In typhoid fever the temperature rises to 102° early in its course, and then by about half a degree or a degree to 104, which point it does not often pass in children, unless there are complications in the lungs or peritoneal cavity. In diseases of the respiratory organs, when the parenchyma of the lungs is affected, the temperature is notably higher than when the mucous membrane alone is affected. In tubercular meningitis there are great ranges, as well as irregularities in the course of the temperature, the maximum recorded is 108.5°, the minimum 95°. When the substance of the brain is affected the rise scarcely ever exceeds 101°. A pulse rate increased to 130 or more per minute and a temperature of 102° is prognostic of meningitis, while a pulse rate of 110 to 120, with a persistent temperature of 104°, points to typhoid fever as the disease.

These general facts will enable you to perceive something of the importance of a study of the temperature. For its full discussion I must refer you to the work of Seguin, and to the works on practice of medicine.

Auscultation and percussion should be practiced in cases of suspected disease of the lung. Auscultation first, and usually you can learn all you wish to know by placing the ear to the back of the chest. The general signs are the same as in adults, except that the vesicular murmur is more distinct or "puerile." By crying and expulsive movements the child can extend the range of dullness fully three inches, by the rising of the lower and abdominal organs against the diaphragm. Remember this, or you will diagnose a pneumonia in a crying child when none exists.

Percussion has not the value in children which it has in adults, because they are more restless, and by their crying obscure all true perception of percussion sounds.

A Case of Caries of the Frontal Bone—Operation—Recovery.

By Ph. Humpert, M. D.

Jan. 13th, 1872, I was called to see C. L——, a man about 45 years of age, of robust frame, and vigorous constitution. He had always been in good health until about two years ago, when, at his former home, through some cause unknown to him, he contracted an inflammation of the left knee joint, which resulted in complete anchylosis.

Four weeks previous to my first seeing him he experienced a dull pain in the left frontal region, which attracted his attention, as he had never before suffered from headache. This frontal headache continued, and was, after some weeks, complicated with considerable swelling and redness of the integuments over the left side of the frontal bone, which soon extended down to both eyelids; at the same time a moderate fever set in. In this condition I first saw him. There was an erysipelas-like swelling over the parts just mentioned, the left eye being entirely closed by the tumefied lids, which caused considerable pain and did not allow of any opening of the eye. Not being certain whether I had to deal with an inflammation of the soft parts (erysipelas), or whether the bone itself was the seat of the lesion, I concluded to fill the most urgent indication, i. e., to reduce the hard chemosis threatening destruction to the cornea by excessive pressure.

Abstracting the stagnant blood by a number of leeches, and applying ice-compresses constantly to the eyelids and forehead, the swelling subsided so much in twenty-four hours that I could open the eye and remove most of the spongy tissue which had gathered around the cornea. But within the same time a fistulous opening had formed in the groove between the upper lid and supra-orbital ridge, discharging a thick, odorless pus. Introducing a probe into the opening, I could pass it upwards about three inches and a little further towards the temporal region. Fully convinced that the frontal bone or its periosteum was the seat of the affection, I made an incision down to the bone, above the outer angle of the orbit, almost three inches long. I found the soft parts indurated and very sanguineous, the external table exhibiting itself as bare, denuded of its periosteum, and of rough, suppurating appearance. From the fistulous opening a probe could be passed through the incision. Cauterizing the surface of the bone as far as it could be reached, with a strong solution of nitrate of silver, I tried to keep the incision open in order to confine the discharge òf pus to the seat of its origin. But in this I utterly failed, the amount of pus discharged through the fistula being diminished only for a few days, and then increasing from day to day, drop after drop oozing out in rapid succession, while all my efforts to keep the incision wound open, were frustrated.

The patient declining any further surgical interference, because, in his opinion, the matter running so copiously should, by no means, be checked, I did not see him again until March 14th, when I found the soft parts over the outer angle of the orbit much improved, especially around the incision cicatrix, presenting very little swelling and redness. But the parts on the left side from the median line and over the inner half of the orbit were in a state of high inflammation, and whenever pressure was made upon them towards the fistula a thick stream of pus was discharged through its opening. From this time on his general health seemed to suffer, owing to the constant drain on his system. But the patient still refusing to submit to a surgical operation, because he did not, nor would not, understand its necessity, I discontinued my visits, until April 19th, when, at the request of his wife, I saw him again, taking Dr. E. W. Schauffler along with me for a consultation. His condition was still worse, showing symptoms of constitutional disturbance foreshadowing a rapid sinking. The frontal region between the median line and the middle of the eyebrow presented a hard infiltrated tumor in a high state of inflammation. The fistulous opening was so far retracted behind the supra-orbital ridge that it was impossible to lead a probe upwards to the diseased bone. Placing the patient under the influence of chloroform, we made an exploratory incision near the median line, three inches long, and after arresting the very profuse hemorrhage from a multitude of almost invisible vessels in the cartilage-like tissues, we introduced a probe and passed it three inches towards the supra-orbital ridge, found most of the bone bare and suppurating, and near the lower edge of the incision we struck a perforation in the external table, of irregular form, and about three-quarters of an inch in its greatest diameter. Through this carious perforation we could pass the probe downwards to the nose and the internal table. We postponed any further operation until, by close observation, we should become convinced of the condition of the frontal sinus, and find out where the profuse suppuration originated, during which time I cleaned the sinus twice daily with a concentrated solution of carbolic acid, besides injecting a solution of nitrate of silver (1 drachm, 1 oz.) every other day. The patient was given the cod liver oil along with syrup of the iodide of iron and quinine.

This treatment was continued until April 28th, when Drs. Schauffler and A. B. Taylor being called in, we submitted him again to a thorough examination, and came to the conclusion that some neorosed particles of bone had to be removed before there would be a chance of his final recovery. The patient being brought under the full influence of chloroform, Dr. Taylor continued the incision made near the median line, to the root of the nose, and made another incision crossing the first at its lower end, and reaching to the middle of the eyebrow. Lifting the soft parts from their bony support, as far as necessary, we found the external table necrosed between the median line and nearly the inside of the eyebrow, forming a square two inches long and one inch wide. After arresting the profuse hemorrhage, Dr. Taylor nipped off ten pieces of dead bone of the average size of the nail of the little finger, thus cutting a hole of the above size. Rounding off every sharp edge of the bone we repeatedly examined the surrounding surface of the external table, and, finding it healthy, united the wound by sutures, leaving a small opening for the escape of pus. The patient suffered very much from the concussion given to the bone with the bone forceps, but after enjoying a few hours' refreshing sleep he was tolerably well next morning. The inflammation following was kept within moderate bounds, and very little surgical fever ensued. All my efforts were now directed to cleaning the frontal sinus from the putrid detritus-like matter which seemed to accumulate at short intervals. Carbolic acid was first used, alternately with nitrate of silver, both in a concentrated solution, but the acid irritating the soft parts too much, was soon substituted by permanganate of potassa diluted with chamomile infusion, which was found to answer admirably. After a few weeks' treatment in this way the sinus proved almost clean of any suspicious matter, while, for the first time, the communication between the sinus and meatus narium medius emptied the injected solution from the sinus. From this time the suppuration was confined to the incision wound, and the edges of the bony opening, the latter growing smaller so rapidly under the healing integuments that after four weeks' uninterrupted improvement I could hardly introduce my little finger. The redness and swelling of the surrounding skin disappeared coëtaneously, and when the wound was entirely closed, leaving only a small groove, the whole forehead assumed an almost natural appearance. The patient became as strong and vigorous as ever in his life, and is now, nearly one year after this most successful operation, still enjoying good health.

The etiology of his case cannot be made out with certainty; syphilis, the most common cause of frontal caries, does not evince any signs of its existence, struma is alike inconsistent with such a vigorous constitution. By my own observation, and by what I know from hearsay, I think it more probable that a long continued "abusus spirituosorum" brought about an alcoholic dyscrasia which finally led to the terrible affection just described.

Correspondence.

Editor Kansas City Medical Journal:

DEAR SIR :—Dr. C. A. Clarkson invites discussion as to the cause of recovery in the case of the mulatto child, two years old, reported by him in his article on " Chlorate of Potassa in Scrofulous Cases," in the December No. of your JOURNAL. I think the difficulty lies in a mistaken diagnosis. From the doctor's report my statement would be: A bad case of mercurialization caused by the administration of "one grain each of calomel and dover's powder every four hours until five were taken." The child may have been scrofulous—probably was—else the mercury would not have affected the whole glandular system so badly.

Possibly the whole course of treatment by means of mercury, iodide of potassium, quinine, etc., may have wrought such changes in the child's constitutional status as to cure the scrofula by the time the mercurialization was cured by the chlorate of potassa with morphine, which we will all admit was a good prescription against the bad effects of mercury.

Very respectfully,   BRYANT GRAFTON, M. D.,
Wyandotte, Kansas.

SELECTIONS.

Practical Medicine.

Relations of Yellow Fever, Malarial Fever, and Malarial Hæmaturia.

BY JOSEPH JONES, M. D.,
Professor of Chemistry and Clinical Medicine, Medical Department, University of Louisiana, and Visiting Physician of Charity Hospital, New Orleans.

I have endeavored by careful observation of the various symptoms, by analysis of the blood, secretions and excretions, and by careful examination of the pathological lesions after death, to unravel the complicated chain of phenomena characteristic of yellow fever and other diseases; and while many facts are unexplained, and much remains to be investigated, we feel assured that the labors which we have pursued unremittingly during the past eighteen months have been at least in the right direction.

The malarial poison induces profound alterations in the constituents of the blood. Under its action, as I have fully demonstrated by the first series of investigations (Trans. Am. Med. Ass., 1859), the colored blood corpuscles are more rapidly and to a greater extent destroyed than in any other disease; the fibrin is diminished and altered in quantity and quality; the albumen is in like manner diminished; the extractive and coloring matters of the blood are frequently increased. The unhealthy hue of the complexion in malarial fever appears to be due to both the destruction of the colored blood corpuscles and the presence of coloring matter in the blood, the deposit of pigmentary matter, and the failure of the liver to separate fully the coloring matter of the bile.

In yellow fever there is no marked or uniform destruction of the colored blood corpuscles. The fibrin is diminished, and to a much greater extent than in malarial fever. There is no tendency to the formation of fibrinous concretions in the cavities of the heart in yellow fever, while the formation of such laminated fibrinous clots is common in malarial fever, and in some cases is the manifest cause of death.

Malaria, by its effects in inducing sudden congestion, and by its depressing effects upon the heart and upon the general and capillary circulation, and by its potent action upon both the sympathetic and cerebro-spinal system of nerves, tends to promote the formation of heart clots, although there is an actual diminution of the fibrin in the blood during malarial fever. In view of the rapid, feeble, intermittent pulse; disturbed, panting respiration; feeble, rapid, fluttering action of the heart; cold extremities, exhaustion of the muscular forces, stupor, wandering of the intellect; inability to control the muscles and acts of excretion ; in view of the sudden onset of all the symptoms in malarial fever; in view of the observations which we have carefully recorded heretofore upon the lesions characteristic of malarial fever, we are justified in asserting that the fibrinous elements of the blood may be deposited in the heart and blood vessels during life in malarial fever, and not only give rise to distinct phenomena, but cause death in cases which would otherwise not have terminated fatally.

It is worthy of observation that in pyæmia and in malarial fever, in both of which diseases there is a more rapid destruction of the colored blood corpuscles than in any other class of diseases, *chills* should characterize both affections, and form the most marked symptom. If such facts do not point out the nature of the cause of malarial fever, they at least sustain the belief that this disease, like pyæmia and yellow fever, is due to the action of a special poison, and not to mere variations of climate and changes of moisture and temperature.

The rapid destruction of the colored blood corpuscles in malarial fever is evident, not only by a comparison of the constitution of the blood in this disease with that of yellow fever, but also by the presence of a larger amount of coloring matter in the urine. As a general rule, the graver the case of malarial fever the more deeply colored is the urine ; while, on the other hand, the reverse is the case with yellow fever. The coloring matter of the urine in yellow fever is due to a great extent to the retention of the biliary matters in the blood and the failure of the action of the liver; while, on the other hand, the deep red and reddish-brown and orange-colored pigments of the urine of malarial fever appear to be derived chiefly from the colored blood corpuscles.

While the presence of the coloring matter in large amount in the urine of malarial fever may be dependent in part upon some imperfection in the excretion of carbon by those organs whose special function is to eliminate this element from the blood, as the liver and lungs, and may, as has been observed by Golding Bird, be connected with some functional or organic mischief of the liver and spleen, or some other organ connected with the portal circulation, at the same time, from a careful consideration of the accompanying symptoms and subsequent post-mortem revelations, we have been led to the belief that in malarial fever the pigment is derived chiefly from the coloring matter of the blood cells, and that its amount may be taken as an index or measure of their destruction. This would be true, whether it comes at once from the blood corpuscles by changes taking place in the mass of the circulating fluid, or by the destruction of the blood corpuscles in the liver and spleen. Certain it is that this pigment is not found in the kidneys, and does not accompany diseases of the kidneys; nor is it thrown off under the action of organic medicines and compounds, drastic and purgative salts, which irritate and even cause disease of the intestines and kidneys. Even tincture of cantharides, when given in such large doses as to cause albuminuria and even blood to appear in the urine, does not cause such pigments as purpurine (Bird), uroërythrin (Heller), or urohæmatin to appear in the urine. In those cases of yellow fever in which we have the greatest irritation of the kidneys, or rather in which there is the greatest structural alteration of these organs, will be found, as a general rule, the lightest colored urine. On the other hand, poisonous metallic salts, which derange the constitution of the *colored blood corpuscles*, and interfere with the *blood-making* or *blood-regulating functions of the liver and spleen*, as the compounds of lead, copper, mercury, arsenic, and antimony, cause even in small doses the appearance of this substance in the urine; and when taken in doses sufficiently large to produce poisonous effects the quantity is greatly increased.

In malarial fever the constituent of the blood which suffers to the greatest and most essential degree is the colored blood corpuscle.

In yellow fever the constituent of the blood which suffers to the greatest and most essential degree is the albumen and its modification, fibrin.

The peculiar action of the poison in the former upon the colored blood corpuscles induces a distinct train of symptoms, and establishes distinct recognizable lesions, characterized chiefly by the deposit of pigment matter in certain organs; while in the latter the poison causes such changes in the albumen and fibrin as to lead to the formation of non-nitrogenous and nitrogenous materials, some of which, as the oil and modified fibrin, are arrested or accumulated in certain organs, as the heart, liver and kidneys.

During the active stages of both yellow and malarial fever, phosphorus and the compounds of phosphorus in the nervous structures, as well as the sulphur and compounds of sulphur in the muscular structures, undergo more rapid changes than in the normal state; and phosphoric acid and the phosphates, and sulphuric acid and the sulphates, appear in increased quantities in the urine when the kidneys perform their offices. The waste of phosphorus and of its compounds in the nervous structures during the active stages of the disease is greater than the supply of these materials through the food. The nervous disturbance and debility characteristic of these fevers, as well as of others, are in a measure due to those rapid changes in the phosphorescent materials of the nervous structures, and especially of the central ganglionic cells.

In many cases of yellow fever, and in that form of paroxysmal fever called *malarial hæmaturia*, the function of the kidneys is impaired, and neither the urea nor the mineral acids are increased in the urine; while at the same time they accumulate in the blood, and exert deleterious effects upon the nervous system and blood. The increase of the urea and of phosphoric and sulphuric acids during the active stages of these diseases should not therefore be considered as anything peculiar, and as at all distinguishing them from other fevers. It is only the tendency to congestion and alteration of the excretory structures of the kidneys that characterize yellow fever. The peculiar intoxication and nervous symptoms, as well as the black vomit of yellow fever, are intimately associated with suppression of the urinary excretion. In many cases I have found the black vomit of yellow fever to *give a strong alkaline reaction from the presence of ammonia resulting from the urea eliminated by the gastric mucous membrane.* I have also detected by repeated analysis *urea in large amount in the brain, heart, liver, spleen, muscles, and blood in yellow fever.* In this disease suppression of the action of the kidneys is more to be dreaded than black vomit, which it often precedes and induces.

The increase of these conditions of the urine is referable to the same cause—that is, increased chemical change—in both fevers, although it is evident that the nature of these chemical changes, and the special constituents involved, may differ in each disease.

During the slow action of the malarial poison, as well as during the active stage of the paroxysm, important changes take place in the liver and spleen which are wholly different from the changes of these organs in yellow fever. In malarial fever, in both the liver and spleen, the colored blood corpuscles are destroyed in large numbers, and the coloring matter resulting from the disintegration of the colored corpuscles accumulate in them, and in conjunction with other changes in the nutritive processes in these organs produce those characteristic alterations of the normal color. In fatal cases cellulose is found in both the liver and spleen, while grape-sugar is absent from the liver. The *bile* also is altered, both in chemical constitution and physical properties.

In yellow fever there is no destruction of colored blood corpuscles either in the spleen or liver, and no deposit of pigment matter, while *oil* is deposited in large amount in the liver, which, together with the bile, impart to this organ a yellow color far different from the *dark slate or bronze color of the malarial fever*. The spleen is comparatively unaltered in yellow fever. Both cellulose and grape-sugar are found in the liver of yellow fever.

That the chemistry of the body is deranged in a definite manner in malarial fever is evident from the changes of the excretions. *During the chill*, and at the commencement of the hot stage, phosphoric acid disappears almost entirely from the urine. As the hot stage progresses, and the febrile action and the heat commence to decline, there is an augmentation of phosphoric acid. The uric acid is either increased or remains at the normal standard during the chill, disappears almost entirely during the fever, and then increases rapidly and rises to a high figure after the subsidence of the febrile excitement, and often continues for days two, three, or even six times more abundant than in the normal state, as I have shown by a large number of observations published twelve years ago.

The sudden variations in the physical and nervous phenomena of malarial fever are accompanied by equally sudden and marked anatomical lesions and changes in the excretions. No such changes in the phosphoric or uric acids are observed in yellow fever. The poison inducing malarial fever acts in a definite manner, and is governed by definite affinities and relationships, and produces a type of diseases distinct from yellow fever. The malaria of the swamps and marshes can only generate paroxysmal fever.

In the vast majority of cases, in malarial fever, albumen does not appear in the urine. This constituent of the blood may, however, be present in the urine in malarial fever under certain circumstances.

1. Its presence in the urine of malarial fever may be due to preceding disease of the kidneys, of the liver, or heart.

2. To the prolonged action of the malarial poison, and the structural alterations induced by it in the spleen, liver, and kidneys.

3. To the congestion of the kidneys from cold, or from the impaction in the capillaries of pigment matter, or from the irritant action of the malarial poison upon the excretory structures in cases which have suffered with repeated attacks of intermittents.

It is the exception to the rule to find albumen in the urine in malarial fever; it is the exception to the rule to find albumen absent from the urine of yellow fever.

Even in those cases where the prolonged action of the malaria has produced profound structural alteration of the liver, consisting in the extensive deposit of black pigment granules within and around the capillaries of the liver, obliteration of many of the branches of the portal system within the lobules, and in the hardening and contraction of the entire organ, albumen is rarely present in the urine. I have examined the urine carefully without detecting albumen in a number of cases of ascites and extreme dropsical infiltration of the lower extremities, produced by the hardening and contraction of the liver in chronic malarial poisoning. I have observed cases, however, in which the kidneys were structurally altered by the malarial poison in a manner somewhat similar to the liver, in which albumen was a constituent of the urine.

A certain proportion of such cases may be referred to the causes which ordinarily lead to structural alterations of the kidneys, as the excessive use or abuse of ardent spirits, and the effects of exposure to wet and cold and extreme temperature; but there are cases of albuminuria which can be explained only upon the supposition that they are due to the structural alteration of the kidneys induced by the prolonged action of the malarial poison. And this condition of the urine is not to be referred to the watery condition of the blood induced by the destruction of the colored corpuscles and diminution of the albumen and fibrin; for the state of extreme anæmia frequently induced by the action of the malarial poison is never attended by albuminuria, unless there be some structural alteration of the kidneys.

In that form of malarial fever characterized by complete jaundice, intense vomiting and nausea, and hemorrhage from the kidneys, which has received different names at different times and in different countries, and which is no "new disease" even in these southern States, the hemorrhage from the kidneys is preceded by congestion of these organs, and is attended with *desquamation of the excretory cells,* and *tubuli uriniferi* of these organs.

Malarial hæmaturia (hemorrhagic malarial fever—new disease—up-country yellow fever,) as a general rule occurs only in those who have suffered from repeated attacks of intermittent fever, or who have been exhausted by a prolonged attack of remittent fever ; and while some of the symptoms, as the nausea, incessant vomiting (and in extreme cases *black vomit*), deep jaundice, and impaired capillary circulation, resemble those of yellow fever, yet there are marked differences, similar to those already indicated, as distinguishing malarial and yellow fever.

The presence of the albumen in the urine of this so-called " malarial hæmaturia " is attended also with the presence of colored blood corpuscles, excretory cells of the kidneys, and the *tubuli uriniferi*, impacted ofttimes with colored blood corpuscles. I have even detected the Malpighian corpuscles containing altered blood corpuscles, and deeply stained by the coloring matter of the blood. As a general rule in yellow fever, the *tubuli uriniferi* are loaded with yellow granular, albuminoid and fibroid matter.

In those cases of malarial hæmaturia which have come under my observation there was evident congestion of the kidneys, attended with desquamation of the excretory cells and coats of the tubuli uriniferi and active hemorrhage. In some of these cases immense quantities of green, biliary fluid was vomited, and the patients died in a state of apparent collapse. As a general rule, suppression of the functions of the kidneys is a fatal sign, and, as in yellow fever, may be attended with convulsions, coma, and delirium. A careful examination of the blood in malarial hæmaturia reveals great diminution of the colored corpuscles and fibrin.

The pathological changes observed after death are characteristic of malarial fever; enlarged, slate and bronze liver, with pigment granules; enlarged and softened spleen, filled with disorganized colored corpuscles and pigment granules; gall-bladder distended with thick, ropy bile, presenting when seen *en masse* a greenish-black color, and in thin layers a deep yellow. As much as one thousand grains of bile of high sp. gr. (1036) have been obtained from the gall-bladder, while in yellow fever not more than one hundred and twenty grains of bile are, as a general rule, contained in the relaxed gall-bladder.

I have thus clearly demonstrated that *malarial hæmaturia* is related to the various forms of true malarial fever (intermittent, remittent and congestive), and in fact is only one of the phases of this fever which may at any time be assumed after the alterations of the blood, liver and spleen induced by the prolonged action of malaria. I have also clearly shown that it is distinct from *yellow fever*, although it may have some symptoms in common, as jaundice, black vomit, and albuminuria.

The treatment of malarial hæmaturia should be conducted upon the same general principles which should guide us in the treatment of *pernicious* intermittent, remittent, or malarial fever; with this addition, that attention should be paid to the condition of the kidneys, and they should be relieved by cut cups and counter-irritation. The bowels should be freely opened by a mercurial (calomel is the best preparation) combined with quinine. Ten grains of calomel and ten grains of quinine is a useful combination. Quinine should be freely given. The strength should be supported by nutritious diet (beef-tea and milk punch), given by the rectum if the stomach will not bear it. Alcoholic stimulants should be used without fear of injury. The action of the skin should be promoted by the hot-air bath and steam bath.

In brief, the *strength must be supported and the paroxysm arrested by quinine; the liver and bowels and portal system must be unloaded; the congestion of the kidneys must be relieved;* and during convalescence the blood must be enriched with pure and nutritious diet and iron, and a gentle action of quinine maintained.—*Amer. Practitioner.*

Chloral; Contra Indications to its Use.

Liebreich points out the following : First—Extended destructive affections of the mucous membrane of the digestive tract ; second—Arthritic conditions are unfavorable, unless the blood first be rendered alkaline; third—In typhus fever, if given at all, it should be in small doses ; fourth—In affections of the circulatory apparatus, particularly in serious valvular and other troubles of the heart, small doses should be used; fifth—hysteria is often a contra-indication, the condition of excitement being sometimes increased ; sixth—Jaundice has been regarded a contra-indication, but this is doubtful. It should never be given in solution stronger than one part to five. · It may be mixed in beer, wine, beef tea, or mucilage ; syrup of orange-peel is preferable. So-called syrups of chloral are solutions in glycerine with sugar. Habitual use does not call for increase of dose, and long-continued use does not impair the general health.—[*Gaz. Hebdom. Dublin Journal.*] Chloral compared with hyoscyamus and bromide of potassium.—Dr. J. A. Campbell has tested these medicines in single doses, a large number of times on fourteen cases of maniacal excitement, and concludes from his observations : First—That both chloral and tinct. hyoscyami are sure sedatives to maniacal excitement; second—That chloral is the more sure hypnotic; third—That chloral acts more quickly than tinct. hyoscyami; fourth— That though bromide of potassium in 60–90 gr. doses is a sedative to maniacal excitement, and to a certain extent, hypnotic, it cannot control severe cases; fifth—That ʒii tinct. hyoscyami, equal nearly 3 grains of chloral.—*Journal Mental Science.*

Hemorrhage from the Bowels in Typhoid Fever under the Cold Water Treatment.

BY DR. C. A. V. WUNDERLICH, of Leipzig. Translated and condensed from the *Archiv der Heilkunde* for the Kansas City Medical Journal.

The writer, who is a son of the distinguished author and clinical teacher of that name, in discussing the question under consideration, gives some interesting statistics concerning the history of Typhoid fever, both before and since the use of cold baths in its treatment.

The hydropathic method of handling these cases, now in vogue in the clinic of Prof. C. A. Wunderlich, is about as follows :

Typhoid fever cases admitted to hospital are usually kept under observation for a day or two before bathing is begun. This is with the view of securing the good influence of rest and systematic nursing, of determining on the gravity of the case, and, sometimes, of confirming or upsetting the diagnosis. If the patient is received during the first week of the disease, or if constipation is present, a dose of four or five grains of calomel is given—otherwise the treatment is expectant in the majority of instances. It having been determined, after the first day or two, that the case is one of at least medium gravity, the cold water treatment is commenced. A bath of the temperature of 64° to 71° Fahrenheit, and of 15 to 20 minutes' duration, is given, whenever the temperature of the body rises during the morning hours to 103°, and during the evening to 104° Fahr., the measurements being made in the rectum. This treatment may, however, be modified by various conditions and accidents.

In those cases that present a continuously high temperature the baths are resorted to earlier than in those presenting a well marked and somewhat prolonged remission. When brain symptoms are prominent, the bathing is commenced without waiting for so great a rise in the temperature of the body. The same thing is true when the fever is complicated with severe bronchitis, or with pneumonia.

The temperature of the baths is maintained at a higher point when the patients are old, emaciated or anæmic; also in case of complication with heart disease, copious diarrhœa, albuminuria, affections of the larynx, pregnancy or menstruation. The duration of the baths is lessened with children or anæmic persons, or on the appearance of feebleness of the heart's action, and, indeed, in the later stages of the disease as a general rule.

During the bath, douches of cold water (usually ice cold) are applied to the head and neck, and these are made the more frequent the more prominent the disturbances of the brain or respiratory apparatus. Between the times of bathing, in grave cases, cold compresses (cloths cooled on ice) are applied to the chest and abdomen. This is done particularly in the earlier stages of the disease and when the remission after each bath is not considerable nor lasting.

The only positive contra-indications to the use of cold baths, according to the practice of the Leipzig clinic, are recent hemorrhages from the bowels, peritonitis, intestinal perforation, and collapse. Under all these conditions, however, except in collapse, the treatment by cold is carried on as far as possible by means of cold compresses and ice bladders.

According to this method the number of baths required daily is commonly from two to four, very rarely more than five or six. In the interval between baths the patients rest quietly and comfortably, and the main object of the treatment by cold—to lower the mean temperature of the day—is sufficiently accomplished.

The number of Typhoid fever patients treated in this way at the Leipzig clinic, from July 1868, to June 1872, was 155. The entire number of Typhoid fever cases treated there during this time was 253—61.3 per cent. therefore were treated with the cold baths. Of those not so treated, the greater part were mild cases, in which the temperature never ran very high—a few were brought in so late as either to be convalescent or moribund, and a few presented the contra-indications specified above.

The assertion of Brand [1] that at least sixty cold baths are requisite for the treatment of a case of Typhoid fever, and that the diagnosis may be distrusted if a less number accomplish the purpose, is opposed by the following statement of the results of the Leipzig method, as described above.

According to Reinhard, [2] during the period extending from 1851 to the fall of 1867 (16½ years) there occurred at Leipzig 213 deaths in 1178 cases of Typhoid fever, a per centage of 18.1. Since the introduction of the cold water treatment in July, 1868, just four years ago, there have been 18 deaths in 251 cases, (this excludes two brought in moribund,) or a per centage

1 Wiener Med. Wochenschrift, 1872, Nos. 6 and 7.

2 Reinhard über Darmblutungen in Typhus abdominalis. Inaugural-Dissertation, Leipzig, 1867.

of 7.2. This ratio of mortality even has been improved upon since a larger proportion of the cases are subjected to the cold water treatment;—thus the years of 1870 to '72 give 173 cases with 8 deaths, or a mortality of 4.6 per cent., hardly a fourth of what used to be lost under the old treatment.

The following is a table of the statistics of other observers on this subject, as far as accessible to the writer:

NAME OF OBSERVER.	RATIO OF MORTALITY.	
	Treated without Cold Baths.	*Treated with Cold Baths.*
Jürgensen (in toto)	15.4 per cent.	3.1 per cent.
" only severe cases	24.4 " "	4.9 " "
Ziemssen & Immermann	30.2 " "	7.5 " "
Hagenbach	26.2 " "	9.7 " "
Betke	17.8 " "	9.9 " "
Merkel	14.2 " "	4.8 " "
Stieler	12 to 15 "	7.9 " "
Goetz	28.7 " "	15.4 " "
Riegel	over 20 "	4.4 " "
Stöhr	20.7 " "	6.6 " "

These are results with which the advocates of the hydropathic treatment have every reason to be satisfied.

Coming to the question of intestinal hemorrhage in Typhoid fever, we learn that according to Reinhard there occurred in his 1178 cases, 57 of hemorrhage, or 4.8 per cent. The reports of Vogel give 4.3 per cent. of hemorrhages, those of Griesinger 5.3, of Louis 5.9, and a number of other observers report about the same proportion, all these being in cases not treated with cold water. On the other hand, the 253 cases treated at the Leipzig clinic since 1868 give 18 hemorrhages, or 7.1 per cent., and 16 of these occurred in the 155 cases treated hydropathically (10.3 per cent). This considerable increase in the proportion of intestinal hemorrhages has very naturally been charged as a direct result of the cold water treatment. The theory of those who hold this belief is that the application of cold to the surface induces a sudden and very decided anæmia of the skin and the parts immediately beneath it; that, as a result of this, an over supply of blood goes to the internal organs, among them the intestines, readily causing hemorrhage, especially from an ulcerated surface.

Dr. Wunderlich defends the cold water treatment of typhus from the charge of being instrumental in causing hemorrhage, on the following grounds:

If the cold baths really brought about intestinal hemorrhage in this way, it ought, in view of the immense number of baths employed, to be of more frequent occurrence than it actually is. Furthermore, the hemorrhage ought to occur during or imme-

diately after the bath, and there ought to be more appearance
of external anæmia and symptoms of intestinal hyperæmia, as
pain in the bowels, etc. The hemorrhages ought not to be
postponed for hours, or even days, after the last bath, as they
are; by which time of course the circulation has had abundant
time to be restored to its proper equilibrium. Among the
18 cases of hemorrhage reported in detail by the author, only
3 occurred immediately after the bath, the balance at periods
of from half a day to several days thereafter. In most of the
latter, one or more bloodless passages from the bowels inter-
vened between the last bath and the hemorrhage.

The period at which enterorrhagia is most liable to occur,
according to Wunderlich, Griesinger and others, is from the
middle of the second to the middle of the fourth week of the
disease, that is, during the period of desquamation. The hemorrhages which took place under the cold water treatment, and
which followed shortly upon the bath, were all during the
second week, a period at which, as is well known, the effects of
the baths on the temperature and circulation of the skin (and
therefore the consequent engorgement of internal organs) is
much less than at later stages of the disease.

The *therapeutical means* used in the Leipzig clinic, on the
supervention of intestinal hemorrhage during typhoid fever,
were the external application of cold (by ice bladders to the
abdomen), and a mixture containing the Muriated Tincture of
Iron. Under this treatment the attack ordinarily yielded without difficulty. In only a few instances subcutaneous injections
of Camphor were employed.

As regards the *results* of intestinal hemorrhage, under the
two kinds of treatment, the testimony is decidedly in favor of
that with cold water. It is well known how grave an accident
this has always been considered, in typhoid fever—how unfa-
vorably it has affected the prognosis, and, in those who survived,
how tedious has been the convalescence. The statistics of mortality in these cases run as follows: Wunderlich, *before* the use
of cold baths, 47.4 per cent. of deaths; Griesinger, 31.2; Murchison, 35.7; Duchek, 71.4, and others in about the same proportion. Among the 18 cases above referred to there were but
two deaths, or 11.1 per cent., and even these did not die as a
result of the hemorrhage.

Dr. W. claims, in conclusion, the following advantages for
the treatment with cold baths, as enabling patients to withstand
the evil effects of these hemorrhages: First—By reducing the
average daily temperature of the body the consuming effect of
the fever is decidedly diminished; Second—The cold baths
have a favorable influence in maintaining the strength of the
patient, as is proved by the facts, confirmed by numerous observations, that during their use consciousness is often restored

where it was lacking, diarrhœa is checked, and, above all, the tongue uniformly becomes clean and moist, giving evidence of a favorable state of nutrition such as was rarely observed in this disease under the old treatment.

Scarlet Fever and Syphilis: A Suggestion.

By EDWARD WOAKES, M. D., Luton.

To most physicians it has occurred to meet with cases of scarlet fever assuming from the outset a distinctly malignant character, at a time when the type of the prevailing epidemic has been of a favourable kind. Under these circumstances, the question must have propounded itself with perplexing urgency —What is it in these exceptional instances that constitutes this virulence? Why should scarlet fever be dreaded as a scourge of worse than Egyptian terror by the members of one family, while in the adjoining house, perhaps, it asserts itself as a comparatively mild ailment?

The following suggestion, towards the solution of this problem, resulted from the observations of four or five distinct epidemics of scarlet fever, and is based upon data supplied by a knowledge of the early medical history of the fathers of the patients. As the result of this historical information in the cases to be briefly detailed, the writer has adduced the conclusion that *their malignity was derived from the circumstance of inherited syphilis.*

CASE I, II.—About twelve years ago a gentleman came under my care with a large Hunterian chancre of the glans penis; and, while under treatment, informed me that he was shortly about to marry. In spite of all remonstrance, he appears to have carried out his intention very shortly after the primary sore had disappeared, and in less than eight months afterwards I was informed that his wife had been confined in a distant town. It was not long before I was called upon to attend this child for very characteristic symptoms of constitutional syphilis; and frequently afterwards did this condition recur, or accompany and complicate every trifling ailment that befel it. In the course of two years another child was born, prematurely, but, by dint of much care, survived, and gave promise of arriving at maturity. Like his brother he manifested the characters of inherited syphilis. A girl was born in due course, also prematurely, but only survived its birth some three weeks. One or two abortions followed, but fortunately no live birth. In the autumn of 1871, during the prevalence of a not remarkably severe epidemic of scarlet fever, the children—having attained the ages respectively of nine and seven years—fell with the disease. The elder one, who was first attacked, rapidly developed symptoms of severe blood-poisoning; stupor, with low muttering delirium, set in within twenty-four hours of the seizure, intense rash, temperature of 105 deg., followed by severe throat symptoms and putrid discharges from the nose and mouth, presaged a fatal issue, which occurred on the sixth day. The second boy then sickened, and though at first with less intensity, he too sank at the close of the first week.

CASE III.—About the same time I prescribed for the child of a groom, aged a little over two years, the subject of scarlet fever. His father, I knew, had a venereal attack three years previously, but, as I did not attend him, cannot testify as to its exact character. This patient progressed favourably for a fortnight, when malignant throat symptoms set in, under which he sank at the end of the third week.

CASE IV, V.—About the period at which the history of the first detailed cases commenced—twelve years since—I treated another patient with primary syphilis. He was apparently well acquainted with the phenomenon, made very light of the occurrence, and ceased his visits long before it was prudent to discontinue treatment. Almost my next introduction to him was in the early part of the present year (1872), when the epidemic of scarlet fever, which had nearly disappeared during the winter, revived and became more general through the inclement spring months. At this period I was requested to see his daughter, about three years old, who was said to be very ill. I then ascertained that of five children born since his marriage this was the only one now living, an infant having died in convulsions, after thirty-six hours' illness, three days previously. This infant, it should be stated, developed a rash a few hours prior to its death, which the friends supposed might be measles, but which there was little doubt was scarlatina. I found the only surviving child in a moribund condition; an ill-developed dusky rash of scarlet fever was diffused over the entire body, sloughy tonsils, enlarged submaxillary glands, stupor, tympanitic belly, and a temperature of 106 deg., left no room for doubt, either on the score of diagnosis or prognosis. This child sank on the sixth day.

It is worth while to note, in passing, that the foregoing were the only fatal cases which came under my observation during the recent epidemic, including a period of nine months.

Here it is necessary to anticipate the objection, that five cases are an insufficient foundation on which to construct any hypothesis sufficiently comprehensive to embrace any large proportion of the special form of disease under consideration. But the purport of this paper being only to communicate instances in which the previous syphilitic history is so clear as to leave no room for cavil, necessarily precludes many cases in which hereditary taint was presumably present, but which lack the essential features of direct medical testimony to the fact. It is hoped that the idea thus broached may lead others to search for indications of constitutional syphilis in the subjects of malignant scarlet fever. The evidences of such infection being not far to seek, it follows that the suggestions now offered will be speedily refuted or as readily confirmed.

The writer must also regret that he is not prepared to advance any satisfactory theory to explain the connection between the two conditions, which he believes he has observed. The facts recorded indicating, as they undoubtedly do, an intense tendency to disintegration on the part of the blood and tissues of these patients, when exposed to septic influences, recall forcibly the recent investigations of Lostorfer, and invest the germ theory of syphilis, as advanced in his researches, with a force of probability, independent altogether of their actual demonstration. But while these views are rightly regarded as at present *sub judice*, the facts so imperfectly submitted in this communication, as well as the inference from them, must be judged on their own merits, and entirely irrespective of any such hypothesis.—*British Med. Journal.*

Hypodermic Injections.

In an article contained in the *Bulletin Therapeutique*, translated in the *Pharmaceutical Journal*, M. Adrian observes that in the preparation of a solution for hypodermic injection, the choice between the normal alkaloid and its salts is not an indifferent one. When medicaments so powerfully active are injected under the skin, it appears necessary to define clearly the relation that exists between the alkaloid itself and its combination with acids. In medical practice sufficient importance is not always attached to this distinction, and instances are sometimes met with where the same doses of hydrochlorate, sulphate, and acetate of morphia, or of hydrochlorate and sulphate of strychnia are prescribed, although the constitution of these various salts assign to them a sensibly different proportion of the active principle that is employed. This will be seen by an examination of the following numbers:

	Crystallized Alkaloid.	Water necessary for solution.
One gramme (15½ grains) of hydrochlorate of morphia contains	0.80	20
Sulphate of morphia	0.76	10
Acetate of morphia	0.86	5
Sulphate of strychnia	0.75	10
Hydrochlorate of strychnia	0.83	8

According to this table, one gramme of acetate of morphia contains a tenth more of morphia than the same weight of the sulphate, and a similar difference exists between the hydrochlorate and sulphate of strychnia. Certain difficulties are also met with in the preparation of the solutions, the solubility of the same salt, probably owing to its state of hydration, varying at different times. Filtration is also requisite in most instances, and the filter absorbs an unknown quantity; in one experiment no less than one-fifth of the total amount of the salt being thus retained. Solutions intended for hypodermic injection, prepared as they usually are, present another defect, namely, the alteration which they undergo after a time. Small fungi are seen to form upon the surface; then the liquid becomes turbid, and gives rise to a copious deposit. M. Adrian's experiments have shown him that the solutions of atropia and codeia are decomposed more rapidly than the others. Also when they are prepared in the cold they change more rapidly than when they are obtained with boiling distilled water. Liquids containing the alkaloids dissolved with the help of sulphuric acid are preserved better than those in which hydrochloric acid is used. Finally, solutions containing glycerine to the extent of one-fifth of the total volume may be kept for a long time without undergoing the least alteration. Based upon these observations, M. Adrian has been led to consider the following conditions to be desirable in the preparation of solutions for hypodermic injections:—1. To use exclusively alkaloids of vegetable origin in a state of purity. These are always well defined, stable, and uniform in composition, whilst their salts vary according to the equivalent of the acid which is used in their formation; and according also as they contain more or less water of crystallization. 2. To use as a vehicle boiled distilled water containing 20 per cent. of glycerine. 3. To give the preference to sulphuric acid diluted in the proportion of one of acid to one of water, above all other acids. 4. To substitute measurement by volume for measurement by weight.— *Practitioner.*

On the Disinfection of Air.

BY A. ERNEST SANSOM, M. D. Lond., M.R.C.P.,
Physician to the Royal Hospital for Diseases of the Chest, and to the Northeastern Hospital for Children.

Few physicians will be inclined to deny that the material poisons of many of the spreading diseases are capable of being wafted by the air from place to place and from person to person, and that in this manner the maladies of infection are in many instances transmitted. In certain diseases—among which may be especially enumerated variola, scarlatina, rubeola, pertussis, pyæmia, erysipelas, and diphtheria—the subjects are centres whence the evolution of disease-inducing particles takes place. It is obvious that complete isolation of an individual, and removal of all the chance of his directly infecting others, are practically impossible; and, even if such were possible, the disease-poison would yet be cast off to attach itself to any surrounding material, still capable of inducing its effects in the future. It would be a measure of the highest importance if the disease-poison, while existing in, or wafted by, the air, could be rendered inert. This is what I mean by disinfection of the air—the rendering inert of the disease-poison which in some infectious disorders is contained in, and transmitted by, the atmosphere.

Many practitioners have attached an importance to the attempt to disinfect the air poisoned by the emanations of those sick of an infectious disease, as a positive duty; and have adopted various methods of carrying it out. Others, however, urge that all attempts in this direction are futile—that it is impossible to disinfect the air.

Let me discuss briefly what is the nature of the material, which I have for convenience called *poison*, that we desire to render inert. It is ponderable, and obeys physical laws. It often remains active for long periods of time, and hence is unaffected by the frequent mutations of the atmosphere; but is so minute as to be entirely undemonstrable by any ordinary direct physical means, and undetectable by the highest powers of the microscope. The diffusion experiments of Chauveau and Sanderson have given convincing proof that in vaccinia, variola, and sheep-pox, the poison is a *solid*, insoluble and indiffusible. This conceded, the area of speculation becomes narrowed; for it is impossible to imagine the material an agent merely organic and gifted only with the properties of inanimate matter. If it be an organic solid, neither soluble nor diffusible, how does it interpenetrate the tissues of the body it so profoundly affects? and how can we explain its immeasurable powers of reproduction? It is not my purpose to trace the analogies of the disease-poison, nor follow the evidence which points to the probability that it is to be endowed with the properties of *living* matter. We must admit one of two views—that it is vitalized, or else it acts by an inexplicable process of catalysis; and if the analogy of other so-called catalytic processes be invoked for the elucidation, we shall find that, as science progresses, these become less and less explicable, on the hypothesis of causation by dead organic material in any state whatever. In fact, I believe it to be true, in the present state of science, that no kind of catalytic change of organic bodies ever takes place without the intervention of living things or their active secretions. I will now turn to the consideration of the methods which have been hitherto adopted for the disinfection of air, and the *rationale* of their action.

First come what are called OXIDIZING DISINFECTANTS.

1. Foremost among these are the alkaline permanganates,

which, when dissolved in water, it is recommended to expose in open vessels to the air of a sick-room, or to diffuse in the form of spray throughout the atmosphere.. The theory is, that these yield up oxygen to the disease poison, and, altering its chemical constitution, impairs its morbific properties. Now it must be remembered in the first place, that these agents are entirely non-volatile. There can be, therefore, no commingling with the air. The particular portions of air which happen to come into immediate contact with the surface of the solution, no doubt have their contained organic particles oxidized; but how feeble a proportion do these bear to the atmosphere of an apartment! The nauseous products of putrefaction, the permanganates have a remarkable power of oxidizing, and thus rendering inodorous; they are excellent *deodorants;* but I have shown them to occupy a very low place both as arresting putrefaction and as killing the low forms of life. A little consideration must show that agents which operate by oxidation only can have but little effect upon the specific poisons of disease. Imagine the minute particles of disease-poison as it is after a long continued relaxation with large volumes of air, this air frequently containing its special oxidizing constituent—ozone; or imagine it commingled with vast bulks of water; surely here are enough conditions for its speedy oxidation and destruction, if it be capable thereof. How insignificant must be the superadded effect of the oxidizing permanganate! In whatever bulk employed, the permanganates do not destroy the microzymes inducing putrefaction, existing in the air superincumbent upon them. From my view, therefore, of the nature of disease-poison, I am justified in concluding that the employment of permanganates as means for the disinfection of air is at once frivolous and futile.

2. Chlorine is also an oxidizing disinfectant; but this stands on higher ground as an air-purifier, because its volatility allows it to come in immediate contact with the particles suspended in the air. It is of a very high value as a deodorant; but its action on fermentation, putrefaction, and on the life of a low organism, is but feeble. I have seen fungi living luxuriantly in and amongst the particles of chloride of lime.

3. Iodine is much more efficacious. It is an oxidizing agent, and hence a deodorant; but it is more—it destroys microzymes, and arrests decomposition. It is of very easy application. If placed in open vessels about a room, it evaporates spontaneously, and is a very useful agent for disinfection of air.

4. Sulphurous acid has also a double action; it is a deodorizer, and hence a deodorant; and it is extremely powerful in destroying the life of low organisms. It has been used (the method of its evolution being merely burning brimstone from a metal plate), and, as the records seem to show, with much advantage.

5. Carbolic acid is a volatile agent, easily diffused throughout the air. It exerts no chemical action thereupon, and thus is not a deodorant; but in my opinion it holds the highest place as a disinfectant proper, for it kills the low forms of life existing in the atmosphere, even when it is present in but small proportion.

Starting with the view that the poisons of spreading diseases are minute particles of living matter, I will now turn to some experimental evidence bearing upon the question of the efficacy, positive and relative, of air-disinfectants. Observation of the effects of different agents, when commingled with the air, upon the low organisms met with in putrefactions, must for the most part offer *a fortiori* evidence; for in many infective liquids the presence of the minutest bacteria cannot be detected. Dr. Sanderson has, however, observed bacteria as the characteristic inhabitants of the infective fluids which transmit pyæmia, "and therefore probably the carriers of infection." Without assuming, however, anything further than that the poisons are *living*, we can, I think, obtain valuable analogical evidence; for the influences which kill bacteria, monads, and germs of fungi, could surely with great probability kill also the minuter particles of living matter constituting the infecting poison.

EXPERIMENT I, *showing that Bacteria and Monads are killed by Air which contains Carbolic Acid.*—A maceration of hard-boiled egg in cold water was observed on the third day after preparation. Multitudes of cylindrical and filiform bacteria and ovoid monads were observed in active movement (magnifying power, 500 and 750 diameters linear). A small drop was placed on a slide, and held for thirty seconds over the open mouth of a flask which contained a little carbolic acid. This was compared with another drop uninfluenced. At first, movements in each case were equally active. In about two minutes in the former, movements became more languid, and soon ceased in many instances. Some, however, continued perfectly active. Experiment was repeated with exposure to carbolic acid for one minute. Monads, at first active, began to move in smaller circles, then merely to revolve on their axes, and finally manifested merely a peculiar vibration. A very marked difference was shown between the exposed and the test-drops; in the former, a large number of bacteria were perfectly motionless. Experiment repeated with exposure for three and five minutes respectively: in the latter case, nearly all were dead. It was evident that the superficial portion was so affected as to render motionless all the bacteria; but in the deeper layer some, though comparatively a very small number, manifested active movement.

Observation has shown me that, whilst the effect of carbolized air upon a fluid capable of putrefaction is to prevent the formation of the usually dense follicle formed by dead bacteria, and to kill those which are superficial, it has no influence upon those below the surface-level, which continue to manifest active movement.

EXPERIMENT II, *showing that the Germs in the Air, which develop into Fungi, are killed by Air which contains Carbolic Acid.*—Two precisely similar glass flasks were taken, and into each was poured some well boiled paste made from wheat-flour. Each was provided with a cork perforated and fitted with tubes for the entrance and exit of air. Over the surface of the paste in A, 500 cubic feet of air were blown by means of a bellows, and then the flask was closed with India-rubber tissue. B was treated precisely similar, except that the air first traversed the surface of six drachms of liquefied carbolic acid contained in another small flask. B was subsequently sealed. The loss of the liquid carbolic acid was half a fluid-drachm. The flasks were then kept in identical conditions. In flask A, after a few days, little islands of mildew appeared; the paste fermented, and disengaged gas-bubbles; and now (thirteenth day) green mould covers the sides, and large masses of white and green mould are on the surface of the paste. In B the paste remains perfectly unchanged, and now (thirteenth day) presents not a trace of fungoid manifestation. These flasks were exhibited to the meeting, and it was manifest that, although more than three weeks had elapsed since their preparation, the paste over which carbolized air had been passed, remained without any sign of decomposition; the other presented a mass of mildew.

I have formerly shown that the appearance of penicillium and aspergillus can be entirely prevented by the presence of carbolic acid in the air supplied to the soil.

EXPERIMENT III, *showing that, whilst the presence of Carbolic Acid or Sulphurous Acid in the Air prevents Putrefaction and the concurrent Development of Living Forms, the so-called Oxidizing Disinfectants fail to prevent either.*—Four small wide-mouthed glass bottles, of similar shape and size, were filled with small cubes cut from a hard-boiled egg. They were then placed each in a small trough, into which was poured the following disinfectant agent in each case: A, commercial permanganate solution (red,) 1½ drachm; B, commercial chloride of aluminium, 1½ drachm; C, pharmacopœial sulphurous acid, 1 drachm; D, crude carbolic acid, 11 drops. Each was enclosed under a glass cover, so as to allow free communication of air both with the open bottle and the free surface of the disinfectant agent; but the cover itself was imbedded in cement, so as to exclude external air. At the end of seven days, the covers were removed, and the bottles containing the pieces of egg were each filled up with distilled water which had been well boiled and then allowed to cool. The covers were then re-applied, and the contents were examined three days afterwards. A (permanganate,) was extremely fœtid, so turbid as to be absolutely opaque, and with a thick pellicle covering its surface. It teemed with small bacteria, and presented many fungoid cells; and the portions of egg were disintegrated; they were in a state of advanced decomposition. B (chloride of aluminium): very fœtid and turbid, rather less so than A. Every drop examined swarmed with small monads and bacteria. The egg-cubes were broken up, and presented signs of advanced decomposition. C (sulphurous acid): Fluid presented no fœtor; was perfectly transparent. The cubes of egg appeared to preserve their shape and condition exactly as when first introduced. On microscopic examination, many fields presented no trace of motile organism; but occasionally a few active bacteria were met with. D (carbolic acid): Fluid appeared almost clear, and the egg-cubes distinct. Very few bacteria presented themselves, usually five or six in a field; they were of unusual length. Decomposition was almost, but not entirely, arrested.

The evidence which I have adduced, I think, fully shows that the presence of certain volatile or gaseous antiseptic agents in the air is sufficient to poison the lowest forms of organisms, to prevent the appearance and development of fungi, and to arrest the putrefaction of organic material. I hope it will be allowed that we who counsel the employment of gaseous or volatile antiseptics for the disinfection of air, do so with the clear understanding of a purpose to fulfil, and a train of analogical evidence that the means are adequate to the end. We believe the subtile poisons of disease to be minute particles of living matter; and that these, given off from a diseased person, can be contained in and wafted by the air. We do not contend that they are equally numerous with the harmless germs of living things which the air normally contains; but they are with them and among them. We show that the presence of antiseptic agents in the air destroys the harmless germs; and we contend that it is probable that it also destroys the disease-germs, which have strong analogical relations with the former, which certainly do not exceed them in bulk, and are probably far more minute than those which are obviously destroyed. As regards the nature of an efficient air-disinfectant, we find that it must be volatile or gaseous, and therefore capable of equable diffusion throughout the air. The non-volatile agents are inert. It is not the action of a chemical agent upon an organic chemical compound which constitutes disinfection, according to our view; but the action of a diffused poison upon the living particles which are suspended in the atmosphere. The agents which I myself believe to be the most efficient are sulphurous acid, iodine, and carbolic acid. Further experience will probably point to many others, but we have these at present to rely upon.

A few words as to the methods of practically employing these various agents :

1. *Sulphurous Acid.*—If the chamber to be disinfected is (*a*) *uninhabited*, all articles capable of being bleached should be removed ; orifices communicating with the external air should be closed, and crevices pasted over with paper. A vessel containing burning sulphur should then be introduced, and the door closed. For the sake of safety from the chance of fire by the overflow of the molten sulphur, it should be kindled upon an iron plate, and floated upon a large vessel containing water. It is convenient to place glowing embers on the plate, and then dust over them flowers of sulphur. If the room is (*b*) *inhabited*, the sulphurous acid must be disengaged in less proportion. Dr. Hjaltelin, who has employed it in small-pox wards, considers that its power of exciting bronchial irritation has been exaggerated, and that patients may be accustomed to it in a high degree. It may be employed in the manner before described ; the flame of the burning sulphur being extinguished by submersion of the iron plate in the water, if the fumes become too powerful. Or, as employed by Dr. A. W. Foot, flowers of sulphur may be dropped upon a heated shovel, and carried about the room. The generation of the gas should be repeated three or four times in the day. It is certain, however, that some persons feel it difficult to tolerate the sulphur fumes.

2. *Iodine* may be used as an air-disinfectant in a very simple manner—first suggested, I believe, by Dr. B. W. Richardson. Solid iodine is merely exposed in glass or porcelain vessels in different parts of the room. The iodine vapour is given off at ordinary temperatures. This is a very efficient mode of attaining a constant disinfection.

3. *Carbolic Acid.*—To employ this agent when the room is (*a*) *unoccupied*—communication with the external air being closed —a quantity of the crude acid should be poured into a strongly heated cup, or upon bricks, and left to vaporise. Subsequently, the floors, ceilings, and, if practicable, the walls, should be irrigated or sprayed with an aqueous solution ; and the floor scrubbed with carbolic acid or coal-tar soap. Or Savory and Moore's excellent vaporiser may be employed, whereby large volumes of carbolic acid vapour may be disengaged. If the chamber is (*b*) *occupied* by the sick, the vaporiser just mentioned, which is so constructed that the liquefied acid falls drop by drop upon a heated plate, should be put in action at intervals twice or thrice in the day. The objectionable odour of the carbolic acid may be greatly masked by its admixture with oil of wild thyme. It is obvious that this method gives off the carbolic acid too powerfully for constant use. The agent, however, is so volatile as to render itself readily available for maintaining a constant antiseptic atmosphere. It has frequently been used in combination

with inert powders for strewing about the room, or has been sprinkled upon cloth or other absorbent materials which have afforded surfaces for its volatilization. These measures, however, have their inconveniences and even dangers; for the strong acid is irritant and caustic, and may inflict serious injury upon those who inadvertently touch it. To obviate the difficulty, I have requested Messrs. Savory and Moore to construct for me an instrument consisting of a piece of canvass in the form of an endless band stretched between two rollers, and dipping into a tin trough to be charged with the acid. By turning a handle at the top, the roller is drawn through the trough, and thus moistened through its whole extent. After it has become partially dry from evaporation, a turn of the handle lifts up a fresh moistened surface. I have used this in several cases, and have found it to act most satisfactorily. I believe, from the data we possess, that in carbolic acid we have the most efficient and most manageable of all agents for the disinfection of air.

Arsenic as a Prophylactic in Rabies.

Dr. Ernest Guisan, in an inaugural dissertation presented to the faculty of Berne, states that though he has arrived at no positive conclusion, he believes, as in cholera, the germ of the contagion in rabies is formed by one of the lowest fungi. The period of incubation extends, upon the average, over five or six weeks. The poison is then absorbed, spreads itself through the body by means of the circulation, and then multiplies indefinitely, producing ultimately irritation of the nervous centres, and especially of the medulla oblongata. Dr. Guisan then enters into the prophylactic treatment of the disease by means of arsenic, and gives the following clinical observations : "A man was bitten on the 24th of June by a mad dog, in the hand ; a girl was bitten at the same time, and shortly after died from hydrophobia. Two days after the accident the man applied to Dr. Guisan's father, who cauterised the wound deeply with potash, and kept the wound open with cantharides. Minute doses of belladonna were given morning and evening up to the 18th July, when the patient had rigors and pains in the body. From this time, up to the 26th of July, the symptoms of hydrophobia became gradually more and more expressed in spite of repeated venesections and the use of calomel and opium. At this date, however, small doses of arseniate of soda were prescribed every four hours (0.003 of a gramme). On the 27th, marked amelioration of the symptoms was observed, which continued till, on the 30th, all danger had passed and complete recovery took place." Dr. Guisan gives another case in which a rabid dog, between the 7th and 9th of June, bit thirteen persons in various towns of the canton of Freiburg. All were recommended to be treated with one-twentieth of a grain of arsenic morning and evening, as a prophylactic measure. Eight submitted to this prophylactic measure, and none were affected. Four declined, or were not allowed, to take the arsenic. Of these four, two remained unaffected, and two died. One began the arsenical treatment, but speedily left it off. She was attacked, but at a much later period, and died. Dr. Guisan not only recommends the internal employment of the arsenic, but that the wound should be dressed with it.—*Correspondenz-Blatt.—Practitioner.*

Surgery.

A Case of Comminuted Fracture of the Leg—Resection and Suture of Fragments.

M. Letenneur, of Nantes, (*Gazette Hebdomadaire*, No. 2, 1871,) reports the following: An individual, aged eighteen, was admitted into the Hotel Dieu of Nantes, on July 10th, 1868. This youth had imprudently placed his hand on a strap which was revolving round a flying wheel. The hand and also the clothes were seized, and the body was jerked into the air, falling at a distance of some metres. On admission the following lesions were made out: A fracture of the surgical neck of the left humerus; a contused wound, occupying almost the whole of the right side of the back, and involving the muscles; a comminuted fracture of the leg, with a wound and protrusion of osseous fragments. The injured limb was placed on a splint, and moderate traction was made on the foot. The anterior tibial artery had probably been torn, as no pulsation could be felt on the dorsum of the foot. The posterior tibial was intact, and this fact, together with the youth and strength of the patient, induced M. Letenneur to refrain from immediate amputation. In order to moderate the inflammatory symptoms, the limb was submitted to continuous irrigation for eight days; it was then dressed with charpie and camphorated alcohol and Labarraque's solution. The traumatic fever was not severe, and the patient retained his appetite. Simple cerate was applied to the wound in the back, and an immovable apparatus to the arm and shoulder. Purulent collections about the fracture in the leg obliged M. Letenneur to make counter-openings. The superior and inferior fragments of the tibia were much notched, and between were splinters of bone, partly imbedded in the muscles. A great number of these were removed, care being taken to separate the periosteum. On putting together these fragments, it was estimated that the bones of the leg would be shortened to the extent of three or four centimetres. There was a constant tendency in the superior fragment of the tibia to project outward, and there was much riding posteriorly on the part of the inferior fragment. As this displacement could not be rectified by ordinary means, M. Letenneur resected the ends of the fragments, and united them by suture. The fragments were thus fixed tolerably firm, and formed in the centre of the limb an internal splint, around which callus might be deposited without any movement being able to destroy this process of reconstruction.

This operation was performed on the twentieth day after the accident. There was then a shortening of about seven centimetres. Considerable though circumscribed swelling then took place at the seat of fracture. Pressure of the finger at this point caused crackling, indicating the rupture of osseous trabeculæ. This swelling at last acquired great proportions and inclosed the fragments and necrosed osseous splinters. M. Letenneur then feared the development of an exuberant callus, hollowed, with abscesses, and constituting an interminable malady. In the month of October the callus had acquired solidity, and the shortening was not more than four centimetres; the limb, therefore, had been elongated by three centimetres. This elongation could not have taken place at the seat of the fracture, as the metallic suture was still in place, and the corresponding fragments were not detached. Finally, in the month of February, the fragments united by the suture became loose, and were then withdrawn with the wire; together they were about eleven centimetres in length. The callus was very solid, but did not then permit the patient to walk. It is remarkable, states M. Letenneur, that the osseous suture applied to bones already dead produced no change in these, and that the openings made by the gimlet had exactly the same dimensions in February as they had when first made. This proves that metallic threads, when they cut gradually through osseous tissues included in the loop of the suture, do so through vital action, and not by mechanical force.

The patient remained in the hospital several months, and after his discharge was readmitted, in order to have some small sequestra removed. When at last he was able to resume his occupation, the shortening did not amount to more than two and a half centimetres. M. Letenneur directs particular attention to the elongation of the bones in this case, which was sufficient to efface the consequences of a loss of substance amounting to seven centimetres. He excludes the sequestra which were removed at a later period, which taken altogether add a length of eleven centimetres. At this period the callus was solid, and its length was not altered in any sensible manner. The elongation, then, in this case, had occurred at the extremities of the bone. In 1856, M. Baizean communicated to the Academy of Science a memoir, in which this phenomenon of pathological physiology was pointed out. In 1869, Langenbeck made a communication on the same subject to the Society of Medicine at Berlin.—*Medical Archives.*

Phosphorus in Skin Diseases.

Of late the attention of the profession has been frequently called to the administration of phosphorus in certain forms of skin disease. The following is condensed from the *Dublin Medical Journal* and the *British Medical Journal*, and presents a résumé of what is known regarding its action:

MM. Husemann and Marane have concluded from their researches that phosphorus, in the uncombined condition, is absorbed into the system, for it can be detected in the liver of carnivora and herbivora by Mitscherlich's process in a few hours after the injection of a very small dose of phosphorized oil into the stomach.

Maelhe confirms this view, and believes that the absorption of phosphorus is due, not to the chemical action of the alkalies in the intestinal juice, but to the fatty matters in the alimentary substances. Hence, in cases of poisoning, it is indispensable to prohibit any food or medicine containing fatty matter.

Voit and Bauer find that fatty degeneration of the organs is produced by phosphorus, even in animals deprived of food and extremely emaciated. The phosphorus diminished both the O taken and the CO_2 given off, but increased the urea excreted. Voit considers that the more rapid degeneration of the liver in acute atrophy is the chief difference between this disease and phosphorus-poisoning. Leucine and tyrosine are among the two first products of decomposition of albumen; at first the fat is formed from the store of circulating albumen, afterwards, as in fasting, from the more firmly combined albumen of the organs, and lastly from that albumen which is essential to the constitution of the cell.

Dr. Vetter says phosphorus prescribed medically has produced acute poisoning, and thinks it should not be ordered in the pure state at all. The treatment he recommends is first an emetic of sulphate of copper, and then oil of turpentine, following this up in a day or two by a teaspoonful of magnesia, now and then.

Eulenburg and Vohl propose charcoal instead of turpentine, as an antidote to phosphorus.

According to Maelhe, it is best administerod dissolved in a

fatty body, which prevents it undergoing change and insures its complete absorption without the inconveniences which attend its solution in ether or chloroform.

Dr. Radcliff's formula for phosphorus pill is : Phosphorus, grs., 6 ; suet, grs., 600; melt the suet in a stoppered bottle, put in the phosphorus, and, when liquid, agitate the mixture till it becomes solid, roll it into 3-grain pills and cover with gelatine. Each pill contains $\frac{1}{33}$ grain of phosphorus.

Dr. Eames, in the January (1872) number, recites a large number of cases successfully treated with phosphorus.

Dr. Burgess was the first in England to call attention to its use in skin affections. He was led to do so from the powerful stimulating effect when given in the stage of collapse in cholera.

Recently, Dr. Broadbent read a paper before the Chemical Society of London, detailing certain cases in which he had given the drug with good effect. Both arsenic and phosphorus belong to the same mineral class, and appear to bear about the same relation to each other in a remedial point of view that they do in their atomic weight. It is a well known fact that many skin diseases will not yield to arsenic, so that if we claim no special curative properties in phosphorus over arsenic, we at least have one more arrow in our quiver. The cases detailed are too lengthy for insertion, but they attest strongly the potency of phosphorus where all else has failed, producing effects that in some instances are truly wonderful.

Dr. Tilbury Fox, in his excellent work on diseases of the skin, recommends it in acute pemphigus and pruritus. Wilson never once mentions its use.

The most convenient mode of administering it, perhaps, is by dissolving 10 grains in an ounce of olive or cod-liver oil and giving from five to ten drops three times daily after eating; or, it may be dissolved in some of the more solid fats, care being taken to stir it constantly while cooling, using the same proportions as before.

It is apt to produce indigestion after being used for some time, such as flatulent eructations, coated tongue, burning in the stomach, etc. When it begins to manifest those symptoms it should be stopped at once and muriatic or nitro-muriatic acid should be administered along with tonic doses of quinine, all fatty articles of food being prohibited for a short time. It is certainly worthy of a more thorough trial than it has yet had at the hands of the profession. But not alone in skin affections does it promise to become useful, but in all those nervous affections for which we have so long been looking to, and leaning on, arsenic for help we may expect the greatest benefit from it. It may in a short time come to be looked upon in those affections in the same light as the preparations of iron are in poverty of the red particles of the blood. Nerve matter is largely composed of phosphorized fat. Now, in administering phosphorus and oil, may we not be giving to the nerve tissue food that it requires, just as in anæmia we, by giving iron, increase the amount of hæmatin in the whole current of the circulation? And more, does'it not point to the organ we are to look to for origin of the local manifestation?

Galvanic Treatment of Bed-Sores and Indolent Ulcers.

Dr. Hammond, of New York, recommends for indolent ulcers and bed-sores, the galvanic treatment, as first suggested by Crussel, of St. Petersburg. He says: " During the last six years I have employed it to a great extent in the treatment of bed-sores caused by diseases of the spinal cord, and with scarcely a failure; indeed, I may say, without any failure, except in two cases where deep sinuses had formed, which could not be reached by the apparatus. A thin silver plate—no thicker than a piece of paper—is cut to the exact size and shape of the bed-sore; a zinc plate of about the same size is connected with the silver plate by a fine silver or copper wire six or eight inches in length. The silver plate is then placed in immediate contact with the bed-sore, and the zinc plate on some part of the skin above, a piece of chamois-skin soaked in vinegar intervening. This must be kept moist, or there is little or no action of the battery. Within a few hours the effect is perceptible, and in a day or two the cure is complete in a great majority of cases. In a few instances a longer time is required. I have frequently seen bed-sores three or four inches in diameter, and half an inch deep, healed entirely over in forty-eight hours. Mr. Spencer Wells states that he has witnessed large ulcers covered with granulations within twenty-four hours, and completely filled up and cicatrizations begun in forty-eight hours. During his recent visit to this country I informed him of my experience, and he reiterated his opinion that it was the best of all methods for treating ulcers of indolent character and bed-sores."

Fall of Temperature accompanying great Wounds by Firearms.

By Paul Redard.

Though the increase of temperature of the body above the standard of health has attracted so much attention, the reverse phenomenon has not been sufficiently studied. Brown-Séquard, however, has shown that, when in illness, or after wounds or poisoning, the temperature falls a certain number of degrees, there is danger of death solely in consequence of the fall.

Long-continued exhausting discharges, want of sufficient nourishment, and hemorrhage, have been observed to produce this fall of temperature; but in a more marked manner has it been seen to follow extensive burns, and to occur in uræmia, in sudden ammonia blood-poisoning, in certain cases of septicæmia, sometimes in chronic peritonitis, in internal strangulation and wounds of the intestines (Demarquay), immediately after apoplectic seizures (Charcot), generally in lesions of the spinal cord and in compression of the brain as in hydrocephalus. Hirtz gives as a pathognomic sign of tuberculous meningitis a fall of temperature coming on at the prodromic period of the malady. A fall of temperature has also been observed after the termination of fever, pneumonia, etc. (the defervescence of Traube), and in various maladies which impede the circulatory and respiratory functions. The administration of digitalis and of tartar emetic has the same effect; alcohol, as a veritable retarder of molecular interchange, causes frequently a considerable fall of temperature; in the acute stage of drunkenness M. Redard has often observed a temperature of 36° (96° 8' Fahrenheit).

Placed during the latter period of the French war—the struggle between the regular army and the Federals—in the ambulances "de la Presse" (in the service of his master, M. Demarquay), M. Redard had ample opportunities of noticing the effect of injuries by fire-arms in lowering the temperature; every time a patient suffering from a grave wound from a fire-arm was observed by him, a lowering of the temperature of the body was found. In most of the cases the injuries had been inflicted by the bursting of shells, but in some they had been caused by cannon balls shattering limbs, and in the instances of the Federals the wounds had usually been received while they were in a state of intoxication. In such M. Redard found a wound produced a much greater fall of temperature than did one of equal extent in men of temperate habits, and in them amputations were most successful. He, therefore, quite indorses the dictum of M. Verneuil, that the prognosis of traumatic lesions, all other things being equal, presents an exceptional gravity amongst subjects addicted to drinking chronically. The author narrates his observations in fifty cases, and concludes his memoir with the following deductions :

" 1. In great injuries by fire-arms fall of temperature is a constantly observed fact.

" 2. Several elements come into play in producing this fall. Amongst the principal we will mention—nervous shock, the excitement of the combat with consecutive stupor, hemorrhage, and, lastly, alcoholism.

" 3. Every wounded man brought into an ambulance with a grave wound, which seems to necessitate an operation, and who shows a temperature below 35° 5' (95. °9 Fahr.), will die, and ought not consequently to be operated on.

"4. Every wounded man in whom a salutary reaction is not produced within four hours, and by whom the reaction is not a direct sequence of the fall of temperature, must be considered as very gravely injured.

"5. Burns give rise to an exceptionally great fall of temperature.

"6. The same is the case in wounds of the abdomen. The fall is the more marked the nearer the wound approaches the stomach.

"7. The diagnosis of penetrating wounds may become less difficult, on account of the characteristic thermometric phenomena to which they give rise.

"8. The state of intoxication in which the wounded are sometimes found favours signally the observed fall of temperature.

"9. Wounds by shells, all other things being equal, produce a fall of temperature more accentuated than those by balls."— *Dublin Jour. Med. Science*, from *Archives Gen. de Med.*

Gynæcology.

Puerperal Mania.[1]

BY FORDYCE BARKER, M. D., Professor of Clinical Midwifery, Bellevue Hospital Medical College.

CASE 1. Mary ——, aged twenty-nine years, born in England, married, entered Bellevue October 5th, primipara ; menstruated last time January 28th. Labor commenced 2 A. M., October 8th, first stage, ten hours ; second stage, three and a half hours ; third stage, twenty minutes. The child, male, weighed nine and a half pounds. Patient was very anæmic, but lost very little blood at the time of labor.

October 9th.—Pulse 84, respiration 18, temperature 99°.

October 10th.—Pulse 80, respiration 20, temperature 98.5°.

October 11th.—Pulse 84, respiration 20, temperature 98°, breasts full. Took two laxative pills, which moved freely twice without pain.

October 12th—Pulse 88, respiration 20, temperature 98.5. Has a large supply of milk ; nurses, by her request, another child besides her own.

October 13th.—7 A. M., pulse 112, respiration 28, temperature 99°. Patient answers questions in an excited way ; stares wildly, eyes very red, but face pale ; says the other women in the ward kept her awake, and were talking all night about her. Lochiæ natural and without odor. Five P. M., pulse 120, respi-

1. From a work on '' Puerperal Diseases '' now in press of D. Appleton & Co.

ration 30, temperature 99.5°. Signs from auscultation and percussion negative. Urinary secretion abundant; no albumen; has been examined every day. No pain or tenderness over the uterus, which is well contracted down in the pelvic cavity. Ordered morphiæ sulph., one-fourth grain.

October 14th.—Patient became so violent in the night that it was necessary to remove her from the ward and to place her in a cell. She talks incessantly and incoherently, using most profane and obscene language. Refuses to nurse her child. Two P. M., seen by Dr. Barker. Pulse 120, respiration 36. Patient so violent and restless that it was impossible to get the temperature. Ordered beef-soup every three hours, and, immediately after each time, quinine, grains 2, muriated tincture of iron, fifteen drops. As the patient had for some twenty-four hours absolutely refused to nurse her child, the breasts were very much swollen and hard; the following to be well rubbed into them : Ext. of belladonna, one ounce, glycerine, two drachms. At eleven o'clock to have chloral hydrate, thirty grains.

October 15th.—Patient is reported to have slept several hours, is very much less violent, but talks incoherently. Answers no questions. Pulse 108, respiration 24. On attempting to use the thermometer, she was apparently frightened, and immediately became much excited. The same treatment to be continued.

October 16th.—Slept a good deal during the night, is much more quiet in her movements, and is very silent generally, but at long intervals talks with great volubility and incoherency. Respiration 28, pulse 112, temperature not obtained. Her condition remained very much the same for the three following days, except that her movements were more strikingly lascivious. Says that she is Mary Magdalen, and calls her nurse sometimes Martha, and at other times Lazarus.

October 20th.—Very quiet, disposes to weep, answers questions. Asks to have the "nasty stuff" taken off her breasts. Pulse 108, respiration 24, temperature 99°. Removed back to the wards. Chloral hydrate reduced to thirty grains at bed time.

October 21st.—Very quiet, taciturn, but occasionally strange. Asked, for the first time, for her child. Cried bitterly when she found the child could get no milk. Wishes to keep it at her breast the whole time. Has revealed to-day, for the first time, that her husband deserted her and left for Colorado with another woman, six weeks before she came into the hospital. From this time she steadily improved. The milk returned to the breasts, and she left the hospital to fill a situation as wet-nurse.

CASE II.—Julia H., aged twenty-two years, single, born in Ireland, pregnant first time. Menstruated last, March, 1871.

During latter part of pregnancy had some swelling of the feet and labia, but clinical examination of the urine negative. Was admitted to the hospital only the day before labor began. Labor began 7 A. M., November 9th. First stage, fourteen hours. Position L. O. A. Second stage, two hours and five minutes. Pains were only moderately severe, but the patient was very nervous and excitable, and seemed to suffer a good deal. Was delivered of a healthy girl, weighing six pounds fourteen ounces, a few minutes after 11 P. M. Placenta came away in ten minutes after delivery of the child. The uterus contracted well, and patient passed a quiet night.

November 10th.—A. M., respiration 24, pulse 68, temperature 100.5°.
            P. M.,   "   27, "   64,   "   100.5°.

Complains of pain and soreness in the chest; occasional pains in the pelvic region. Ordered Magendie's solution of morphia, ten drops.

November 11th.—A. M., respiration 26, pulse 76, temperature 100°. Had a chill, beginning at 12 M., which lasted two hours, followed by high fever and sweating. During chill, complained of pain in lower part of back and abdomen.

Seven P. M.—respiration 32, pulse 148, temperature 104°. No sweating, no pain, except when she moves. Slight tenderness in inguinal region. Breasts swelling, no tympanites. Ordered tincture aconite, three drops every hour, until three doses had been taken. Quinine, five grains every third hour.

November 12th.—9 A. M., respiration 32, pulse 104, temperature 105°.
        12 M.,   "   32, "   108,   "   105°.
        3 P. M.,   "   30, "   108,   "   104.7°.
        9 P. M.,   "   30, "   132,   "   104°.

No pain or tenderness in abdomen. Occasional pain in back running down the legs.

November 13th.—A. M., respiration 32, pulse 112, temperature 105°.
       6 P. M.,   "   32, "   100,   "   101°.

Aconite stopped, continued quinine. Patient feels much better. Has a little milk in the breast for the first time this evening.

November 14th.—A. M., respiration 28, pulse 84, temperature 101.5°.
            P. M.,   "   30, "   112,   "   103.7°.

Has a little cough and some soreness in the chest, with a little pain in the lower part of the abdomen when she coughs. Some tympanites. Ordered Magendie's sol. of morph., ten drops, and turpentine stupes to abdomen.

November 15th.—A. M., respiration 25, pulse 84, temperature 101.3°.
            P. M.,   "   24, "   96,   "   102.5°.

No pain, very little tenderness. As bowels have not moved for two days, ordered laxative.

November 16th.—A. M., respiration 30, pulse 96, temperature 104.3°.
            P. M.,   "   30, "   104,   "   103.5°.

Nervous and excited, no pain, bowels moved, tongue cleaner.

November 17th.—A. M., respiration 30, pulse 96, temperature 102°.
                P. M.,   "   30, " 109,   "   104.5°.

Patient very excited. Has some pain in the stomach and over uterus. Vaginal examination reveals tenderness on both sides of uterus, but no swelling or hardness. Quinine, five grains every third hour. Poultices to abdomen.

P. M.—Patient very wild. Has been nervous and hysterical ever since her confinement. Has been suffering great mental anxiety for fear that her misfortune would be known. Yesterday a friend visited her in the hospital, and told her that her seducer was married. Since then she has acted very strangely, at one time crying bitterly, then begging the nurse not to heed her, and then again becoming very violent, and has delusions as to her identity. Bowels open. Bromide of potassium half a drachm, at bedtime.

November 18th.—A. M., respiration 30, pulse 84, temperature 100.5°.
                P. M.,   "   26, "   96,   "   103.5°.

Patient more quiet, with less delusions, but still very excitable. Slept most of the night. No pain.

P. M.—Complains of pain and tenderness over the hypogastric region. Ordered poultice to abdomen and a suppository of watery extract opium, one grain.

November 19th.—A. M., respiration 30, pulse 96, temperature 101.5°.
                P. M.,   "   34, " 112,   "   104.5°.

Patient rational. Pain and soreness in right iliac region.

P. M.—Ordered tincture of aconite root, two drops, every second hour.

November 20th.—A. M., respiration 30, pulse 72, temperature 99°. Patient feels better. Aconite stopped.

P. M.—Respiration 36, pulse 95, temperature 102.7°. Patient very nervous. Says she did not sleep last night. Pain, tenderness, and some tympanites of the abdomen. Turpentine stupes, and chloral hydrate, thirty grains.

From this date until the 25th the condition of the patient did not essentially change. She slept well under the influence of the chloral hydrate.

November 25th.—Respiration 22, pulse 88, temperature 97.8°. Patient feels well. No pains, and appetite good. She subsequently left the hospital perfectly well.

The cases you have just seen belong to a class which occurs very frequently in this hospital, or to quote from the "Obstetric Clinic" of Prof. Elliot: "In Bellevue we receive a great many cases of puerperal mania, on account of the fact that so large a proportion of our pregnant women are unmarried primiparæ, and because others of the poorest classes, who cannot be controlled at home, are sent to the hospital."

Since I have been connected with this hospital, now seventeen years, I have had one or more cases of this malady every time I have been on service, with but one exception. In the autumn of 1861, the first year of our international war, I had five cases of puerperal mania; in the spring of 1862, three; in the autumn of 1863, following the great riots in this city, I had six cases; and during my present service (November and December, 1870) I have had three. I estimate the ratio of puerperal mania to the whole number of cases of labor to be one in eighty in this hospital.

Now, I beg you to notice the wonderful contrast in frequency of this malady here as compared with the statistics of other hospitals in other parts of the world. Scanzoni states that in Wurzburg, in forty-six years, there were five cases of puerperal mania out of 7,438 confinements, that is, one in 1,587. He also states that the records of Prague, from 1835 to 1848, show that, in 23,347 cases of labor, there were nineteen instances of puerperal mania, one in 1,228.

In the lying-in wards of St. Giles's Infirmary, one series of cases gives one case of puerperal mania in 1,888 of labor, and another series one in 950. McClintock and Hardy 6,634 cases of labor, give eight cases of puerperal mania, one in 816. Johnston and Sinclair (Dublin Lying-in Hospital) twenty-six cases of mania in 13,748 of labor, one in 528. At Westminster General Lying-in Hospital there were nine cases in 3,500 of labor, or one in 383. At Queen Charlotte's Lying-in Hospital there were eleven in 2,000, or one of mania in 182 of labor.

Now, let us look at the statistics of this disease from another point of view.

Marcé, who has written in some respects the most complete essay on this subject that has appeared, finds that the records of "Public Institutions for the Insane" show that about eight per cent. of the insane are due to puerperal causes.

The statistics of Scanzoni, taken also from public institutions, some being the same as those of Marcé, also furnish a percentage of about seven per cent. as resulting from puerperal causes.

Dr. J. B. Tuke, whose valuable papers on the statistics of puerperal insanity, published in the *Edinburgh Medical Journal*, in 1865 and 1867, are the most suggestive of anything that I have read on the subject, gives the following statement: "Between January 1, 1846, and December 31, 1864, there were 2,181 female cases of insanity treated in the Royal Edinburgh Asylum;" of these 155 were so-called puerperal cases, making a percentage of 7 to 1. You see that there is a remarkable agreement of authorities in regard to the proportion of insanity from puerperal causes compared with all other causes as shown by the statistics of public institutions.

Another point, not to be overlooked, is that, in private practice, probably one-half of the patients recover from this malady without entering a public institution. My own experience would lead me to suppose the proportion to be much greater than this.

At all events, I think it may reasonably be assumed as proved that fully seven per cent. of the insanity which occurs among women, in civilized and Christian communities that support insane hospitals, are due to causes connected with child-bearing.

Let me say here that the term puerperal mania is ordinarily used very loosely. Dr. Tuke in the papers that I have just alluded to, remarks with truth and great force : " In works on midwifery and mental diseases, we find the several forms of insanity which occur during pregnancy, follow parturition, and supervene on lactation, all arranged under the common head of puerperal mania. This, with regard to the first and third divisions, is of course a misnomer, a contradiction in terms; and it seems rather curious that it should have been so long adhered to, more particularly as it tends to confuse and almost stultify deductions made from the few statistics of puerperal mania of which we are possessed. For instance, any comparison, drawn between any given number of labors and any given number of so-called puerperal cases, must lead to erroneous conclusions, if the insanity of pregnancy is confounded with puerperal mania, or if, as is the case, the anæmic insanity of lactation is confounded with either."

The 155 cases of Dr. Tuke are classified by him as follows :

Insanity of pregnancy --- 28
Puerperal insanity--- 73
Insanity of lactation--- 54

The first group, insanity of pregnancy, thus bearing a percentage of 18.06 on the total of 155 ; the second, puerperal insanity proper, 47.09 ; and the third, insanity of lactation, 34.08.

The insanity of pregnancy and the insanity of lactation are more frequently met with by the alienists and the physicians to insane hospitals than by the obstetrician proper; and, although my remarks will be chiefly confined to the subject of puerperal mania, I will say a few words in relation to each of these forms, and also another form, the delirium of labor.

INSANITY OF PREGNANCY.—It is a matter of common observation that, in women of certain temperaments, habits, and education, pregnancy so modifies the nervous system as to produce morbid appetites, changes of temper and disposition, sometimes moral perversion, unnatural sadness, or a settled conviction of impending death.

The diseases of the female sexual organs often produce these reflex disturbances to such a degree as to cause real insanity,

and, as it is important for all of you, who are to have the respon-
sibility of the health and happiness of the families committed to
your charge, to understand this, I will take the present opportunity to say a few words on this too neglected subject.[1]

*   *   *   *   *   *   *   *

But pregnancy is a physiological process, and the instances
in which the reflex disturbances from this condition result in
insanity must be rare. I have seen but two such cases, and in
both the evidence of hereditary predisposition was conclusive.

One of them had repeated attacks of epilepsy, the first year
of her menstrual life, and the other had been previously insane, but was supposed to have entirely recovered more than
two years before her marriage. In both cases the insanity was
permanent. I am indebted to others, and especially to Dr.
Tuke, for what I have to say in regard to this form of insanity.

Esquirol found hereditary predisposition in more than one-
third of the cases that came under his observation (5 in 13).
Dr. Tuke's statistics show that primiparæ are by far the most
liable to this malady, "a circumstance which might have been
expected when we take into consideration the moral exciting
causes, anxiety, and dread of the coming event, which exist to
a greater degree in the inexperienced woman." The type of
the disease is almost invariably melancholic. In the twenty-
eight cases of Dr. Tuke only two are reported as characterized
by mania, and he believes that, in those rare instances where
mania occurs, it will be found that the patient has previously
been the subject of insanity in that form.

In no form of insanity is the suicidal tendency so well
marked as in the melancholia of pregnancy.

In the earlier stages it seems very amenable to treatment.
Cases are on record in which the insanity of pregnancy is said
to have disappeared with labor, but this does not seem to be a
common result. If the mental symptoms disappear before or
at the time of confinement, there is a marked tendency to re-
currence for a longer or shorter period of time. These cases
seem to be particularly benefitted by treatment in the special
hospitals for insane, as the assurance of protection, the regular-
ity, amusement, and employment, alone to be found in an asylum—above all the freedom from domestic anxiety and the mis-
applied sympathy of relatives—in a large majority of cases are
productive of the best results.

THE DELIRIUM OF LABOR.—This is sometimes excited by the
force and intensity of the pains in the second stage. It has been
described by Velpeau, Cazeaux, and more fully illustrated by
the late Dr. Montgomery, of Dublin, and I suppose most who
have been long in practice have occasionally met with such

1. This portion of the lecture "On Insanity caused by the Disease of the Female
Sexual Organs " was published in the Boston *Gynæcological Journal*, May, 1872.

cases. Since the common use of anæsthetics in midwifery, these cases must be very rare. I have seen but one case in the past twenty-four years, and, as this was a very peculiar one, I will briefly relate it:

The patient, a lady of high culture and remarkable good sense, without the slightest hysterical tendency that I have ever been able to discover, awoke about five in the morning, near the end of her first pregnancy, shrieking, "I am drowning, I am drowning!" and jumped from her bed. The nurse, who was sleeping in the hall bedroom adjoining, with the door standing open, and the husband, who occupied the back-chamber, rushed in and found her tearing about the room in the most frantic manner, screaming incessantly, without listening to a word said to her. I was immediately summoned, and, living very near, was with her in a very few moments. I had previously ordered chloroform in anticipation of her labor, but it required the united efforts of her husband, nurse, and other servants of the house, to hold her sufficiently quiet for me to bring her under the influence of the anæsthetic. I overwhelmed her with the chloroform as speedily as possible, and then, on making an examination and finding an arm protruding from the vulva, I delivered at once a living child by turning. The after-birth speedily followed, the binder was applied, and she was placed in a dry bed before she awoke. She had, undoubtedly, been aroused from her sleep by the rupture of the membranes, discharge of the waters, and escape of the child's arm. It is quite certain that less than an hour elapsed from the time of its occurrence until she awoke quite calm and quiet from the sleep of the chloroform, yet one can easily understand the emphatic declaration of her husband that this hour was an eternity to him. By my urgent injunctions no allusion to the incidents of her first labor has ever been made before the patient, and she has often expressed her surprise to me that her only recollection of it should be that, on awakening she saw her mother holding a baby.

INSANITY OF LACTATION.—I have seen but seven cases of this type, and these were all in consultation. All recovered from the insanity, but two died within a few months after I saw them, from phthisis. All of these were cases of Melancholia. As I before remarked, the physicians to insane hospitals see these cases much more frequently than obstetricians. It is essentially due to anæmia of the brain. Dr. Tuke says that when mania occurs it is of an evanescent nature, violent while it lasts, but not associated with the obscenity observable in puerperal mania. Both forms, mania and melancholy, are readily curable when taken in time.

PUERPERAL MANIA.—The insanity which first shows itself during the puerperal period is most properly called puerperal mania, for this is the type of the disease in a great majority of cases. In Dr. Tuke's table, fifty-seven out of the seventy-three cases of puerperal insanity were cases of mania. It is my belief that, if the cases which occur in private practice during the first fortnight after labor, and which either recover within a couple of weeks or pass into the stage of dementia or melancholia, and form no part of hospital statistics, could all be aggregated, it would be found that fully 90 per cent. have the original type of mania.

Again, puerperal mania is generally manifested during the first two weeks after confinement, and by the end of the month the patients have recovered or the disease has passed into a different type.

Puerperal melancholia rarely, if ever, is developed until the latter half of the month, and these, being the most intractable, are the cases which are most likely to be transferred to insane hospitals. At least this is the result of my observation.

Puerperal mania is the form which obstetricians have most frequently to deal with. In some few rare cases, it is suddenly developed without any forewarning symptoms, but, in by far a larger number, there are very characteristic prodomic symptoms, sometimes continuing for a few days and in other instances only a few hours before the explosion. There is generally an unusual excitement of manner, although, in a few, a morbid melancholy air first attracts attention. A sudden aversion is displayed toward those who have been before best loved; an excessive loquacity, or an obstinate silence, weeping or laughing equally without a motive, a morbid sensibility to light, to noises, to odors, a suspicious, watchful expression of the eye, and sleeplessness, are symptoms, which, occurring in a woman who has been confined within ten or fifteen days, indicate an impending attack of puerperal mania. There are often muscular movements of the eyelids, the face, and the hands, very much resembling the appearance of one on the brink of delirium tremens. Indeed, the general symptoms are often wonderfully like those which are characteristic of the beginning of delirium tremens, and in the case of the wife of a medical friend, which I will presently relate to you, a painful suspicion existed in the mind of her husband at first that the real disease was delirium tremens.

Then there are certain symptoms which very generally characterize the moment of attack, but are usually of short duration. The facial expression is very peculiar, and, having once been seen, will always be remembered. The features are drawn, pallid, and the cheeks and forehead are covered with little drops of perspiration, and the whole air of the expression is unsettled, indicative of fright or fury.

But, when the malady is fully developed, the patient becomes very boisterous and noisy, incoherent in her language and in her gestures. She stares wildly at imaginary objects in the air, seizes any word spoken by those near and repeats it with "damnable iteration," clutches at every thing and every one near her, throws off all covering, jumps from the bed, and even the most refined and religious women, when possessed with the demon of puerperal mania, will scream out oaths and obscenity with a volubility perfectly astounding. Erotic manifestations occur in a majority of cases. Masturbation is sometimes noticed, but I believe, as Dr. Tuke suggests, that this is more the result of a wish to allay than excite irritation. Nearly one-half of these cases manifest a suicidal tendency, but rather as a sudden impulse than a settled determination.

While many of these symptoms are very like those of delirium tremens, the physical symptoms are in striking contrast with those of this disease. The patient is pale, cold, clammy, with a quick, small, irritable pulse; the features are pinched, at times almost collapsed-looking. There is usually great muscular weakness, with now and then a momentary spasmodic display of unusual strength.

I wish especially to urge it upon your attention that other grave diseases may exist in a latent form, coincident with the mania, the symptoms of which are masked by the mental symptoms. In this hospital, one patient has died with pelvic peritonitis, another with pneumonia, and a third with pericarditis and endocarditis, and in neither was the disease suspected until revealed by the autopsy. All recent authors agree that phrenitis connected with puerperal mania is excessively rare.

PROGNOSIS.—This involves the three questions of the duration of the disease—the mental recovery—and the recovery of the health. Dr. Tuke says: "Puerperal mania of itself does not kill, and when you have to combat it alone, not only death is not to be dreaded, but, in the very large proportion of cases, a return to sanity may be prognosticated. It is, perhaps, *the* most curable form of insanity. This statement is made advisedly, but does not extend to those cases which are placed under asylum treatment as a *dernier ressort*." As to duration of the disease, in some, but comparatively few cases, it entirely disappears in a few days. I have been struck with the fact that in all cases that I have seen, where the mania has followed puerperal convulsions, the duration of the mania has been limited to three or four days, and the patient has speedily recovered, or she has died within this period. I only mention the fact, without attempting to offer any theory to explain it.

In a majority of cases, the mania gradually subsides within a period of three weeks, more frequently earlier, and is followed by a condition of partial dementia, with some delusions, especially as regards personal identity. These gradually disappear, leaving a kind of intellectual barrenness, like one waking from a dream. From this condition you may confidently hope for ultimate recovery. In some cases, the malady is prolonged two or three or more months; but, if beyond six months, the chances of recovery are very small. When death is the result, it is almost invariably due to some associated disease, as peritonitis, or cellulitis, pneumonia, and in some very rare cases phrenitis, and the fatal result usually occurs in a few days.

CAUSES.—Among the predisposing causes, hereditary tendency is the most prominent, especially traceable to the female side of the family much more frequently than to the male. This was proved to exist in twenty-two of the fifty-seven cases of Dr. Tuke. Esquirol 1 in 2.8; Marcé 24 of 56; Helftt, of Berlin, 51 in 131.

The next cause which I shall mention as predisposing to this malady is dystocia. In the seventy-three cases of Dr. Tuke (including both mania and melancholia), the labor was complicated in twenty-three. Dr. Tuke remarks: " The various irregularities of labor doubtless operate in different ways, those where the suffering has been long continued depressing the nervous system directly, those in which large quantities of blood have been lost producing anæmia of the brain, and, in the case of the child being still-born, a moral shock acting on the mind naturally predisposed to this affection." I will add, to those causes that I have mentioned, anæmia and eclampsia. Moral causes are no doubt among the most frequent of the predisposing causes, but they are also

EXCITING CAUSES.—It is my firm conviction that mental emotions constitute the exciting cause of puerperal mania infinitely more frequently than all other causes combined. The relative frequency of puerperal mania is just in proportion to the susceptibility to the influence of emotional causes. In Wurzburg the proportion of cases of mania to the whole number of confinements was one in 1,487; in Prague, one in 1,228. It is not strange that Scanzoni, studying the malady in this field, should regard the frequency of mania as exaggerated, at the same time that he admits that hospital records probably do not accurately represent the relative frequency in private, as it is notoriously more common in the well-to-do classes. Now, while this is undoubtedly true in Scanzoni's field of observation, the exact reverse of this statement is true with us. I have visited the lying-in hospitals of Wurzburg, Prague, Munich, and many others in Germany, and I have conversed with Scanzoni on this very subject. From him I learned that, with most patients in these hospitals, there is no sacrifice of domestic ties or social position in going to the hospital, but, on the contrary, they are every way better off than when out of the hospital.

They have never before been so well cared for. For most of them, there is no stigma of disgrace in being there, and no consciousness of moral wrong or loss of position among their associates by becoming a mother without being a wife. Among the lower classes in some parts of Germany, I believe it is considered a perfectly legitimate business for girls to become pregnant to qualify themselves for the position of wet nurse and earn some money. There is, then, an entire absence of those moral causes of puerperal mania which exist in tremendous force in this hospital, as I will presently show you.

Then contrast the difference in frequency between the patients in the lying-in wards of St. Giles's Infirmary, where in one series there was one case of mania in 1,888 confinements, and the patients of Queen Charlotte's Lying-in Hospital, where there was one of mania in 182 of labor.

Now, mark the difference between the moral condition of the patients in this hospital and those whose statistics I have given. A large majority of patients in our lying-in-wards are of foreign birth. They have come to a new country, many of them leaving friends behind, with the hope of improving their condition, and many are disappointed in this respect. A large proportion, probably more than one-half, are unmarried. It is impossible to ascertain the truth on this point, for many represent themselves as married and deserted by their husbands, and some of these are subsequently found to be single. But this very deceit shows a moral sense on this point. Then many, who have been seduced and abandoned by their seducers, prefer to die in the hospital rather than have their disgrace known to their relatives. In addition to this, I am well convinced that our climate has a marked influence in developing the nervous susceptibilities of Europeans who come here. Then, again, there is no part of the world where the lapse from virtue in women is so severely punished by social ostracism as in New England, and she contributes her quota of poor girls who rush to a great city to hide themselves, and are at last driven to the hospital as their only resource.

Now, in view of all these facts, I think that you will agree with me that, if statistics ever prove anything in regard to the causes of disease, they prove that moral emotions are the great exciting cause of puerperal mania.

I will mention a curious fact that has occurred in my experience. Since 1855 I have seen thirteen cases of puerperal mania in the wives of physicians, nine in this city, and four in the adjoining cities. All but one were primiparæ. It has struck me as very extraordinary, that so large a number should have occurred in one special class, and I think this is the probable explanation : Every one of these were ladies of education, and more than usual quickness of intellect, and, beginning a new experience in life, and having access to their husbands' books, they probably had read just enough on midwifery to fill their minds with apprehensions as to the horrors which might be in store for them, and thus developed the cerebral disturbances, just as any other moral emotions may.

Some authors have sought to show that the exciting cause of puerperal mania was to be found in the peculiar state of the sexual system which occurs after delivery. Others would make anæmia and exhaustion the principal exciting causes.

Others, again, and most prominently the late Sir James Simpson, regard puerperal mania as especially due to a toxæmic condition of the blood, and as most frequently associated with albuminuria. Sir James Simpson suggests that "mental emotion probably acts intermediately on the mind by its morbific agency on the body." He also says that, "he has only seen one instance of late years attributable to such a primary depressing mental cause, and in this case the urine was highly albuminous, as it is usually found in puerperal convulsions." Many others have seemed to adopt the views of Prof. Simpson in regard to the influence of albuminuria in developing puerperal mania. Dr. Foster Jenkins, of Yonkers, published an interesting case of puerperal mania in the *American Medical Monthly*, 1857, in which Prof. Alonzo Clark and himself found albumen abundant in the urine; the patient was treated mainly for albuminuria, and recovered. My late friend, Prof. Elliott, was disposed to regard albuminuria as a prominent element in causing puerperal mania, but, of the five cases of puerperal mania reported in his "Obstetric Clinic," not one was associated with albuminuria.

As for myself, since the suggestions of Sir James Simpson were first published on this subject, I have been on the constant watch for albuminuria in every case of puerperal mania that I have seen, and I have found it associated with so small a proportion of the cases, that I am compelled to regard it, when present, as simply a coincidence and not a cause. To adopt Prof. Simpson's remarks relative to anæmia and exhaustion as a cause, I should say the alleged cause is very, very often present in practice without the alleged effect following. The theory at best, if applicable at all, is applicable to a very limited number of cases, and affords no more satisfactory explanation of the origin of the disease than does the more general statement that puerperal mania results from the peculiar state of the sexual system which occurs after delivery.

[*To be continued.*]

On Pyæmia.

By Edward Copeman, M. D., F. R. C. P., Senior Physician to the Norfolk and Norwich Hospital.

The occurrence of several deaths, during the past year, in our hospital from pyæmia (so called), induces me to bring before you a few remarks upon the subject, in the hope of being able to elicit, by discussion, some more definite ideas as to the nature and treatment of this very unsatisfactory disease. When fully established, it appears to resist treatment, and cannot be controlled; at least, such is the conclusion at which most of us must arrive from what we have recently seen. One of the theories with respect to its causation, is that pus is absorbed into the blood, poisons this vital fluid, and leads to secondary deposits in some of the important organs of the body. But my own firm belief is that the theory is without foundation, and that pus is never absorbed into the blood. Pus is a bland fluid, unirritating, healing, and the result of one of the natural processes for the cure of inflammation. In a healthy individual, I do not believe that pus ever does any harm unless it be confined in a space which will not give way to it, and make injurious pressure upon other organs. How often do we see abscesses, when favorably situated, become absorbed without any injurious consequences; how disappointed we feel if wounds which do not heal by the first intention do not suppurate; we augur from it that the patient's strength is not sufficient to allow the formation of pus, and we have little hope of recovery. How often do large wounds, after operations of various kinds, continue to suppurate for days, weeks, or months, and we have no fear of ill consequences arising from it so long as the pus is *laudable*. My own opinion is that the true cause of pyæmia, which I would rather call cacæmia, rests in the constitutional condition of the patients, and that the disease is by no means confined to cases of surgical operations. We all know that the blood always contains the ingredients, so to speak, of pus, and can at any time form it when nature seems to require it for the cure of inflammation. Whenever inflammation occurs, there is what Cullen called *spasm of the extreme vessels;* and this frequently results in the formation of abscess. In inflammation, whether acute or chronic, active or passive, there is congestion of the inflamed part, and generally there is matter formed for the relief of this congestion. We see it in the formation of matter in the glands under the jaw in scarlet fever, in the skin in small-pox, in the liver in hepatitis, in the lungs in certain forms of pneumonia, in the prostate gland, in the eyeball, in the cellular tissue in carbuncle and erysipelas, in various organs in different kinds of fever—in fact, in any part attacked by inflammation; and I look upon the occurrence of secondary abscesses after operations as instances of partial stagnation of the blood (passive inflammation) when it is in an unhealthy state, and unable, for want of nervous influence, to eliminate any morbid elements it may contain. This is especially the case with respect to the liver, which contains more blood than any other organ, and so abscesses are often found there; and I do not think it would be stretching the point too far if we were to say that the same thing occurs in the lungs in cachectic subjects, where a number of small abscesses form around passively inflamed bronchial tubes, eventually forming tubercle, the absorption of the watery part of the pus, leaving the residue in a semi-solid form. I do not say that this is the *rationale* of the formation of tubercle, but it seems to me as reasonable as any other, and quite in accordance with the ordinary rules of morbid phenomena terminating in abscess.

Speaking of an accumulation of blood in an organ—the spleen, for instance—and the consequent formation of tubercle, Dr. Carswell says: "In one cell you may perceive simply the blood coagulated; in another, it may be coagulated and deprived of its coloring matter; and, in another, converted into a mass of solid fibrin, having in its centre a small nodule of tubercular matter." And speaking of the fact that the superior and posterior portion of the upper lobe is the spot in which tubercles, if any exist, are almost sure to be found, and where they first begin to suppurate and soften, he adds that, in his experience, there is no deviation from this rule, except when some other portion of the lung may have been the seat of an inflammatory attack, which has determined the priority of tubercular disease in that portion." (Sir T. Watson's *Lectures*, 5th edition.)

We must all have remarked the extraordinary similarity of the symptoms leading to death in all diseases which lapse into a typhoid state, whether from fevers or inflammations, or after surgical operations; the rough dry tongue, the rapid feeble pulse, the relaxed skin, obtuse sensorium, colliquative perspiration, panting breathing, powerless muscles, relaxed sphincters, and very frequently vomiting of green or grumous fluid. Surely some common cause for this must be at work; and that cause I deem to be a morbid condition of the vital fluid—the blood; and this whether attended with secondary abscesses or not. There can be no doubt that this fearful condition of things may be very much promoted, if not actually caused, by air impregnated with a *materies morbi*, and that pure air and good ventilation are most desirable and necessary adjuvants in the treatment; but it should be borne in mind that such cases occur often in great malignancy in country districts as well as in hospitals; and as far as my experience will guide me, a well regulated hospital is more healthy than many country villages during the prevalence of an epidemic which terminates in what we always used to call typhoid symptoms.

A word as to treatment in cases of so-called pyæmia after surgical operations. No doubt the principal points are good nourishing food, good pure air, and such an amount of stimulants as will *strengthen* without *accelerating* the pulse; such as will *diminish* and not increase the rapidity of respiration. But surely medicine may lend its aid, and in some instances may turn the scale in the patient's favor, although the general state of things appears almost hopeless. I do not intend to weary you with any long detail of the treatment in general; there are several points so evident to all of us as to the use of tonics, aperients, and opiates, that they need not be enumerated. But there is one agent to my mind of great value, and which I have seldom seen fairly tried in cases of pyæmia after surgical operations. Once, on passing casually through a ward at the hospital, I met with Mr. —— at the bedside of a patient who was apparently in a hopeless typhoid condition, and in whom, if he had died, it would have been probable, from analogous cases, that internal abscesses might have been found. I suggested to him the use of oil of turpentine. Mr. —— replied that he thought the man would die; and, as he had nothing more to suggest for his relief, he would order him turpentine. The man recovered. You all know the analogy which exists between cases of puerperal fever and surgical fever; and I have at various times, shown to you how beneficial the use of turpentine has been in many of the former cases; indeed, in this and the adjoining counties, there is a rapidly growing belief in its efficacy; and I have been requested by several practitioners, conjointly, as well as individually, to make my further experience known to them. This I intend to do shortly; and shall bring before this Society a sufficient number of cases, in addition to those I have already published, to corroborate the opinion I have so often expressed about it. Now, why should we not give it a trial in these cases of surgical fever? The patients die as it is. Why not make the experiment of turpentine? Speaking of fever, the late Dr. Graves (the greatest physician of his day) remarks as follows: "I have seen people's lives saved by a few doses of the oil of turpentine, and have watched its tranquilizing effect on the nerves with pleasure and surprise." The mode in which he gave it was: oil of turpentine, 1 drachm, castor oil, 1½ drachm, water 1 ounce; to be taken every sixth hour. I should very much like to find that our surgeons are disposed to give this valuable medicine a trial when their operated patients are *going*, not only when they are *gone*, into a typhoid state. Should it succeed, well; should it fail, no harm could have arisen from putting it to the test of experience in cases which almost always die without it—*British Med. Journal.*

Phytolacca Decandra in the Treatment of Inflammation of the Mammary Glands.

By G. W. BIGGERS, M. D., La Grande, Oregon.

The following cases are stated as the *result of my experience* only with the remedy in question, and I trust that others may try it and report the result.

CASE I.—Mrs. H., on third day after labour with her second child, mammæ commenced swelling, from an accumulation of milk. Did not see her until the symptoms were so urgent that there could be no mistake about the commencement of an abscess.

I pursued the antiphlogistic treatment, both general and local, until there was no promise of improvement; on the contrary, the case was continually getting worse. I then prescribed fluid ext. phytolacca decandra, gtts. xx, every three hours, in water. A very marked improvement took place in twelve hours, and in thirty-six hours the patient was well. There was also a suppression of the lochia, which was also re-established.

CASE II.—Mrs. B., whose child died a few hours after its birth, was attacked, after the secretion of milk took place, with inflammation of the mammary glands, from over distension, and had the milk withdrawn very regularly, yet the case continued worse, threatening an abscess. I prescribed fluid ext. phytolacca decandra, gtts. xx, every three hours. Marked improvement in ten hours, and a complete recovery in thirty-six hours. There was also a suppression of lochia in this case, which was re-established with the cessation of the mammary inflammation.

CASE III.—Mrs. G., at the fourth month of pregnancy, was attacked with inflammation of both mammæ, severe pain, swelling, and very great heat, with severe rigors, amounting to a distinct chill. I prescribed fluid ext. phytolacca decandra, gtts. xv, every three hours, in water. The symptoms all subsided, and the patient fully recovered within forty-eight hours with no other treatment.

I have used the remedy above named in many other cases of mammary inflammation, and it has never yet failed in a single case.

The preparation used was Thayer's fluid extract, for the reason that the plant does not grow in this State. A tincture from the green root would, I think, be more reliable.—*Am. Jour. Med. Sciences.*

THE KANSAS CITY

MEDICAL JOURNAL.

Editorial.

We take pleasure in announcing that in future the name of Dr. GEO. HALLEY will be associated with the editorial management of the JOURNAL.

The senior Editor cordially welcomes such able assistance in a task which, by reason of the constantly increasing demands of professional duty, was becoming truly onerous.

It is believed that, by this addition to the editorial force, greater variety as well as increased vigor will be added to the JOURNAL, and that its circulation will be correspondingly extended.   E. W. S.

A Simple and Efficient mode of using Plaster of Paris Splints.

Of late there is much in the current medical literature on the use of and mode of applying plaster of Paris splints. Now, while they all have points of merit that none will deny, there are points to which very serious exceptions can be taken.

Dr. Du Bois, in the Dec. number of the *Western Lancet*, strongly recommends the application of a thin roller bandage into which has been well rubbed finely powdered (dry) plaster. After the fractured ends of bone have been brought into apposition he dips a roll of prepared bandage into a basin of water and applies it to the limb. In a few moments he puts on a second and third, and so on till from five to seven thicknesses of bandage have been applied.

The objection to this mode of using the plaster of Paris is that, after putting it on in the way described, it has to be cut with a strong knife or scissors, if any change in the size of the limb occurs. And 2d, that in order to apply it with sufficient firmness to prevent displacement of the fragments, from the equal pressure on all sides of the limb, it is apt to strangulate it.

A method I have been practicing with the best result is a slight modification of that described by Langenbeck. I take an old piece of army blanket, when I can get it, and out of it cut two *double* splints, one for each side of the limb. Take the leg for example: I fold the blanket double, put the fold along the median line of the back of the leg, bring the two free edges round to the median line in front, cut now so as to leave a margin in front. I prepare a similar splint for the opposite side in the same way. With a strong double thread I now sew the two splints together along the crease made by the fold that came to the median line of the back of the leg. I now with the help of an assistant or assistants have the limb drawn off the couch and properly supported, extension being constantly kept up.

I prepare my plaster in the ordinary way. If there are local injuries I dress them with an antiseptic wash, cover with a small piece of lint wet with a solution of carbolic acid, take the inner portion of each of my lateral splints, bring them firmly round to the front of the leg and fasten either with pins or by sewing. Having an ordinary roller at hand I now with my hand or with a dish bathe the single layer of splint, saturating it fully with the plaster. As soon as it begins to show symptoms of *setting* I bring up my second fold, rapidly spread some more plaster over it and apply the roller firmly, but not very tight, and my splint is as solid as stone in twenty minutes.

The advantages I claim for it are these: From having a seam in the median line of the back of the leg there is a narrow space on which there is no pressure, so that if swelling sets in there is no danger of strangulating the limb. My roller is not starched and I can at any time remove it after the plaster has dried, and by simply cutting the sewing down the back of the leg I can remove the splint without the least trouble, dress any wounds of the soft parts and re-apply without injuring the splint in the least. If the limb begins swelling relief can be had at once, or if the limb is swollen when it is applied, the bandage can be tightened as occasion may require. Compound fractures are put up in this way by Langenbeck and allowed to remain till they show symptoms of requiring dressing. When it is done the same splint is again applied, being removed from time to time as occasion may demand. I have used this splint and find it superior to all other methods. The plaster of Paris splint is applicable to a large majority of fractures of the extremities and deserves more attention from the profession than it has yet received. Let those who are skeptical on the subject try it and we predict for them the happiest results.   G. H.

Meeting of the State Medical Society.

The Medical Association of the State of Missouri holds its next annual meeting at Moberly, on Tuesday, the 15th of April.

So far as we know there are no questions of an ethical nature to come up for dispute, nor any matters of general policy that need to occupy much time. Let us hope then that those who meet at Moberly will do so with the desire and the fixed resolve to discuss medical science in some of its more practical aspects.

The reports of the regular Committees, if made, will give us enough to talk about; and besides these there will be papers read by other members. Let us be determined to consider these—to make time for them—and resolutely to stamp down all attempts of miserable malcontents who would transform the meeting of the State Society into a police court for the hearing of their petty grievances, or into a State laundry for the washing of their local soiled linen.

To some of our brethren who happen to live in towns or counties where there is no medical Society in active operation, and who are on that account a little reluctant about presenting themselves for membership to the State Society, we would say, emphatically, you are the very ones who will be most welcome. Come, by all means. If you have an interesting case to report, jot down the particulars and bring it along; if you have a question to propound, come with your question, and you may start the most valuable discussion of the meeting. Come, anyhow, and help us to talk, or at least help us to listen.

Reviews.

THE MICROSCOPE AND MICROSCOPICAL TECHNOLOGY. A Text-book for Physicians and Students. By Dr. HEINRICH FREY, Prof. of Medicine in Zurich, Switzerland. Translated from the German and edited by George R. Cutter, M. D., Clinical assistant to the New York Eye and Ear Infirmary. Illustrated by 343 engravings, and containing the Price Lists of the principal Microscope makers of Europe and America. From the Fourth and last German Edition. 8 vo., pp. 658. New York; Wm. Wood & Co., 1872.

The fact that, during the few years that this book has been before the German-reading public, four large editions of it have been sold, speaks more loudly in its praise than can any word of the reviewer. Dr. Cutter deserves, and will receive, the thanks of all workers with the microscope, in this country, for having placed within their reach so valuable and practical an aid and guide to their labors.

The first three "sections," or chapters, of the book treat of the theory of the microscope and describe a number of the instruments most generally in use. The theory is set forth briefly but clearly, and without any waste of time in the discussion of abstruse, and as yet unsettled, questions in the science of optics. The fourth chapter, (32 pages,) entitled "Testing the Microscope," contains much information of especial value to any one who is about to purchase an instrument and who desires to do so intelligently; it also tells the student how to test the magnifying power of his microscope, and gives a list of test objects, with accurate diagrams of the same. The nature, advantages, and method of handling "immersion lenses" are explained; the author tells "what he knows" about European opticians, and the translator closes the chapter with an interesting "history of the microscope as an American instrument," and very sensibly advises Americans to buy instruments of home manufacture.

More than one-third of the entire work is taken up with teaching the "Use of the Microscope," including, of course, the preparation of microscopic objects, methods of staining, drying, freezing, injecting, mounting, etc.

The remaining pages are occupied with a description of the microscopic appearances presented by the various tissues and organs of the body. By far the larger space is given to depicting the normal or physiological appearance of the tissues, rather than those conditions which are the result of disease. This may be a disappointment to some ardent pathologists, but will be a source of great satisfaction to the majority of students, who have been too much in the habit of finding in other works on microscopy, as well as on medicine generally, elaborate descriptions of abnormal appearances, with nowhere a picture of the same tissue or organ in a state of health.

61

This portion of the work contains a large number of most admirable engravings, which we should like to see adorning the pages of our text books on Physiology.

One omission is observable : the entire absence of any allusion to animal or vegetable parasites.

Taken as a whole, the treatise of Prof. Frey is one of the most interesting and valuable of the many German works recently put into the hands of the English-reading public, by American enterprise.

The work of the translator has been done faithfully and well; the typography and binding are elegant; and the book is not too bulky for convenient use.. S.

THE PATHOLOGY, DIAGNOSIS AND TREATMENT OF DISEASES OF WO-
MEN, INCLUDING THE DIAGNOSIS OF PREGNANCY. By GRAILY
HEWITT, M. D. Lond. F. R. C. P., Prof. of Midwifery and Diseases of Women,
University College, and Obstetric physician to the hospital: Honorary Fellow
of the Obstetrical Society of Berlin; Vice-President of the Obstetrical Society
of London. Second American, from the third London edition, revised and
enlarged. With one hundred and thirty-two illustrations. Philadelphia:
Lindsay & Blakiston, 1872.

This is one of the most valuable of the really good books which sometimes come to us from across the waters; a value which is not lessened by the fact that it was written abroad, and therefore, like works on the practice of medicine, liable to the suspicion of having a more or less limited adaptation, since the diseases and conditions pertaining to the diseases of women are for the most part the same throughout the civilized world.

As might be expected by those familiar with the first American edition, this revised and greatly enlarged work is a thorough and reliable exponent of the latest and most enlightened views on these subjects. Dr. Hewitt, however, has not stopped here. He is a well-known enthusiast in his particular department of medicine, and has long borne the reputation of being a most competent, careful, and conscientious observer of facts, a vigorous writer, and a merciless critic. The present volume has afforded him ample opportunity for the exercise of these qualities, as well as the elaboration and systemizing of his long-digested theories respecting Mechanical force in its relations to Uterine Pathology.

The "mechanical system of uterine pathology," as our author calls it, is indeed an important feature of the book, and if his etiological views of a large class of pathological conditions are to be received, must necessitate a practice in which local stimulation and depletion in many cases of *unsuspected* change of form, or dislocation of the uterus, shall be subordinated to mechanical supports.

We cannot close this brief notice of a book so full of original thought: so thoroughly comprehensive in detail : and, withal, so thoroughly practical, without an acknowledgment of grati-

tude to the author for his convincing argument that well-
marked cases of retroversion and anteversion are extremely
rare, flexion being to a greater or less degree almost inevitably
associated with them.   S. S. T.

A HAND-BOOK OF POST MORTEM EXAMINATIONS AND OF MORBID
   ANATOMY. By FRANCIS DELAFIELD, M. D. 8vo., pp. 376. W. Wood &
   Co., N. Y., 1872.

When we look over the numerous works issued from the
medical press, we are inclined to believe that the ground has
been all occupied, and that no new subject can be found on
which to write, and yet, every once in a while, some work
fresh from its author's hands comes to us, so completely novel,
that it at once raises the question : Why was this subject not
written on before ? Such is the case with the work whose title
is at the commencement of this notice.

It occasionally happens that the physician is called on to
make a post mortem examination, for medico-legal or other pur-
poses, and in such case, unless his attention is directed to all
necessary points of inquiry, some are often overlooked. This
is just the work he needs for such an emergency, it gives him
plain directions how to proceed with the operation, and what
points to look for as he proceeds, while the method to be followed shows that the writer has been long practically familiar
with his subject.

It affords us great pleasure to give this work our highest
recommendation.   J. L. T.

LESSONS IN PHYSICAL DIAGNOSIS, by ALFRED L. LOOMIS, M. D., Etc.

This small volume again comes to us in a new dress, still
keeping the place, however, which it at first took, viz : a primer,
or First Book of Lessons in Physical diagnosis. To be an
exhaustive work it makes no pretensions, nor to take the place
of such works as Walsh or Da Costa. But it is the work of all
others for the student setting out in the pursuit of the elemen-
tary principles of physical diagnosis. To the busy practitioner,
also, it is of signal value; from its concise form, short, terse
style, and methodical arrangement, he can at any moment refer
to it, and find without trouble just what he wants. We heartily
recommend it to the profession.   G. H.

A MANUAL OF QUALITATIVE ANALYSIS. By ROBERT GALLOWAY, F. C. S.
   12mo., pp. 142. Philadelphia: Henry C. Lea, 1872.

This work having reached a fifth edition has fully received
its " imprimatur," but it seems strange to find the " operations"
required to be performed and the reagents to be used, described
at the end instead of the beginning of the book. Many of the

practical little points, the learning of which saves a student so much time, are omitted, such as the use of a small glass rod in pouring solutions from one vessel to another; the care in washing precipitates always to begin at the upper edge of the filter, and, so going round, wash the precipitate at last down to the bottom; the use of the filtering bottle to save time where the filtrate is not needed, etc., etc.

In spite of these little deficiencies, however, the Manual is a practical and valuable work, which has already made for itself an excellent reputation. ·   J. L. T.

Miscellany.

THE MEDICAL ASSOCIATION OF THE STATE OF MISSOURI holds its next annual meeting at Moberly, beginning on Tuesday, the 15th day of April.

The Committee on Scientific communications consists of Drs. S. S. Todd, of Kansas City, Joseph Smith of St. Joseph, and J. C. Bernard of Hainesville. Gentlemen having papers which they desire to present before the Society will please forward them to the chairman or to any member of the Committee a few days before the date of the meeting.

Nothing has yet been heard from the committee of arrangements (Dr. J. C. Tedford, Chairman), with regard to any reduction of railroad fares to delegates. If arrangements of this sort can be made, they will undoubtedly be announced in due season.

UNIVERSITY OF THE STATE OF MISSOURI.—A Medical Department of the University has been organized, to be located at Columbia, Boone County. Four M. D.'s and one Ph. D., all residents of Columbia, thus far constitute the Faculty. They only propose to give a half session this year.

THE LATEST SELL ON JOHN BULL.—The London *Chemist and Druggist* says: "An American friend assures us that in South Bend, Indiana, they use small packages of quinine for change. As every body takes quinine they look upon it the same as legal tender, and it passes without difficulty."

A WARNING TO THE LADIES.—The following is clipped from the New York *Tribune:* "Coroner Keenan was asked yesterday by Dr. C. P. Russell, Registrar of the Bureau of Vital Statistics, to hold an inquest on the body of Elizabeth T. Church, wife of Dr. E. P. Church, of 629 Ninth Av., who died Jan. 5th 'from abscess of the right lung, caused by an injury inflicted with a wire by the deceased during an attempt to procure an abortion upon herself.' Dr. Russell stated that an autopsy by Prof. T. G. Thomas, of the 23d St. Medical College, had 'revealed the presence of a wire about twenty inches long,' which had passed upward through the peritoneal cavity and penetrated the lung."

PERSONAL.—Dr. C. B. Brigham, of Boston, has been decorated by the Emperor of Germany with the Imperial Order of the Crown, for his services to German and French soldiers in the hospitals at Nancy.——Prof. Agassiz has been elected one of the eight foreign associate members of the French Academy of Sciences, to fill the vacancy caused by the death of Sir R. I. Murchison.

CZERMAK.—Died, recently, at his house in Graz, Prof Czermak, Dr. of Medicine, and the director of the Styrian Insane Asylum, a man well known in the medical world for his extensive and original labors in the department of Psychology.

VOLTAIRE'S DEFINITION OF A PHYSICIAN is: "An unfortunate gentleman expected every day to perform a miracle; namely, to reconcile health with intemperance."

BOOKS AND OTHER PUBLICATIONS RECEIVED.

THE PATHOLOGY, DIAGNOSIS AND TREATMENT OF THE DISEASES OF WOMEN, including the Diagnosis of Pregnancy. By Graily Hewitt, M. D., Lond., F R. C. P., etc.,etc. 2d American from the 3d London edition. Philadelphia: Lindsay & Blakiston, 1872.

CLINICAL LECTURES ON DISEASES PECULIAR TO WOMEN. By Lombe Atthill, M. D., Univ. Dub., etc., etc. 2d edition, revised and enlarged. Philadelphia: Lindsay & Blakiston, 1873.

Annual Report of the Surgeon General, United States Army, 1872.

Treatment of the Phimosis produced by Chancroidal Ulcers. By R. W. Taylor, M. D. New York: F. W. Christern, 1872.

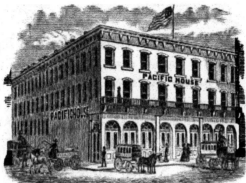

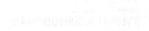

Lightning Source UK Ltd.
Milton Keynes UK
UKHW012331061118
331891UK00010B/944/P